PROXIMAL HUMERUS FRACTURES

EDITED BY
MICHAEL A. WIRTH, MD
PROFESSOR AND CHARLES A. ROCKWOOD, JR, CHAIR
DEPARTMENT OF ORTHOPAEDICS
UNIVERSITY OF TEXAS HEALTH SCIENCE CENTER
SAN ANTONIO, TEXAS

SERIES EDITOR
THOMAS R. JOHNSON, MD
ORTHOPAEDIC SURGEONS, PSC
BILLINGS, MONTANA

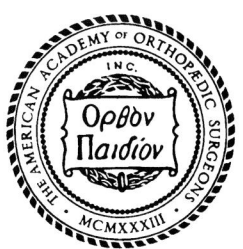

American Academy of Orthopaedic Surgeons

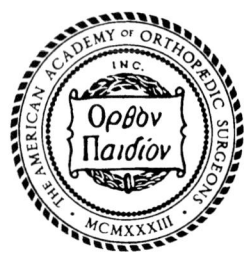

Proximal Humerus Fractures

Published by the
**American Academy of Orthopaedic
Surgeons**
6300 North River Road
Rosemont, IL 60018
1-800-626-6726

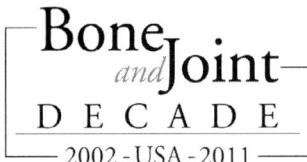

CONTRIBUTORS

Matthew T. Boes, MD
Shoulder Fellow
Department of Orthopaedic Surgery
Beth Israel Medical Center
New York, New York

Frances Cuomo, MD
Chief, Shoulder and Elbow Service
Department of Orthopaedic Surgery
Beth Israel Medical Center
New York, New York

Andrew Green, MD
Associate Professor
Department of Orthopaedic Surgery
Brown Medical School
Providence, Rhode Island

William N. Levine, MD
Vice Chairman and Associate Professor
Associate Director, Center for Shoulder, Elbow, and
*   Sports Medicine*
Department of Orthopaedic Surgery
Columbia University Medical Center
New York, New York

Steven B. Lippitt, MD
Associate Professor
Department of Orthopaedics
Northeastern Ohio Universities
College of Medicine
Akron General Medical Center
Akron, Ohio

Margaret J. Lobo, MD
Chief Resident
Department of Orthopaedic Surgery
Columbia University Medical Center
New York, New York

Peter J. Millett, MD, MSc
Shoulder/Sports Medicine
Steadman Hawkins Clinic
Vail, Colorado

Maryangela Moutoussis
Research Assistant
Department of Orthopaedic Surgery
Beth Israel Medical Center
New York, New York

Jon J.P. Warner, MD
Chief, The Harvard Shoulder Service
Department of Orthopaedics
Massachusetts General Hospital
Boston, Massachusetts

Michael A. Wirth, MD
Professor and Charles A. Rockwood, Jr, Chair
Department of Orthopaedics
University of Texas Health Science Center
San Antonio, Texas

CONTENTS

PREFACE

The Rubicon River of Northern Italy formed a boundary between Cisalpine Gaul and Italy, the crossing of which by Julius Caesar in 49 BCE was regarded by the Roman Senate as an act of war. For many orthopaedic surgeons, the management of proximal humerus fractures is one of the most challenging problems in orthopaedics, and treating some of these injuries is comparable to crossing the Rubicon. Results can be immensely satisfying or incredibly frustrating, and the journey irrevocably leads down a path ending with great praise or severe disappointment.

Over the past decade, continued interest in the shoulder has led to an increased understanding of its basic science and pathophysiology, which has led to improved diagnosis and treatment of shoulder girdle fractures. Despite these advances, the results of both surgical and nonsurgical management as determined by validated outcome measures suggest that these results are often only satisfactory at best. To this end, we offer this monograph in hopes of improving patient outcomes and increasing surgeon satisfaction with these often perplexing injuries.

This monograph owes its strength and appeal to a number of factors, not the least of which is the forum of eminent authorities who have been assembled, individuals with long and successful clinical experience managing fractures of the proximal humerus. It is the goal of this monograph to provide a classification of proximal humerus fractures that is both comprehensive and relevant. This monograph also emphasizes the importance of sound clinical assessment and addresses the current concepts in closed treatment. It discusses minimally invasive surgical techniques such as percutaneous pinning and more traditional methods of open reduction and internal fixation of two- and three-part fractures. The monograph also includes a discussion on humeral head replacement arthroplasty for complex fractures and fracture-dislocations of the proximal humerus. Finally, it addresses the late sequelae of these fractures, ranging from refractory shoulder stiffness to malunion and nonunion.

I would like to offer special thanks to the senior authors for enlightening us, teaching us, and showing us a better way. But most of all, a debt of gratitude is owed to all of the contributors for the most important contribution of all–the priceless gift of their time in making this monograph possible. Finally, I would like to thank the staff of the AAOS Publications Department for bringing this project to fruition.

Michael A. Wirth, MD
Editor

CHAPTER 1

CLASSIFICATION AND CLOSED TREATMENT OF PROXIMAL HUMERUS FRACTURES

MARGARET J. LOBO, MD
WILLIAM N. LEVINE, MD

Fractures of the proximal humerus account for 2% to 4% of upper extremity fractures and 5% of all fractures seen in emergency departments.[1] Treatment decisions are based on the mechanism of injury, the patient's health and activity level, and the fracture pattern. Most nondisplaced or minimally displaced fractures are treated nonsurgically, whereas displaced fractures typically require surgery. Determination of appropriate treatment requires a functional understanding of the anatomy of the proximal humerus. Classification systems should provide treatment algorithms and predict outcome if they are to be used successfully. In this chapter, we review classification systems and closed treatment options for proximal humerus fractures.

EPIDEMIOLOGY

The incidence of proximal humerus fractures varies with sex (three times as many in women as in men) and age, similar to the incidence of fractures of the femoral neck. There is a rapid increase with age, which is twice as fast in women as in men. Only avulsion fractures of the greater tuberosity deviate somewhat from this pattern.

The more displaced fractures have a tendency to occur later in life.[1]

Seventy-five percent of all proximal humerus fractures occur in patients older than age 60 years.[2] In these patients, the primary mechanism is low-energy trauma, such as a fall on an outstretched hand.[3] Risk factors for proximal humerus fractures in the elderly include poor bone quality, impaired vision and balance, medical comorbidities, and decreased muscle tone and strength.[4] Predictors of fracture in women who do and do not have osteoporosis have been studied. Factors independently associated with an increased rate of fracture include a recent decline in health status, a previous fall, type I diabetes mellitus, infrequent walking, and several indicators of neuromuscular weakness such as inability to stand with feet in a tandem position for more than a few seconds.[5,6] Most of these fractures are nondisplaced and have a good prognosis with nonsurgical management.

High-velocity trauma, such as a motor vehicle accident, is the primary mechanism of fracture in younger patients. Seizures and electrical shock are potential indirect causes of proximal humerus fractures. Fractures resulting from high-velocity trauma are often more severe, with associated dislocations and soft-tissue disruption and almost always require surgical intervention. In young patients, every attempt should be made to restore anatomy and preserve native bone.[7]

ANATOMY AND BIOMECHANICS

Anatomy

The proximal humerus comprises the articular head, the greater and lesser tuberosities for insertion of the rotator cuff, and the shaft. The shaft connects with the head at the metaphyseal flare just below the tuberosities; this is the surgical neck. The anatomic neck is above the tuberosities between the articular surface and the articular capsule. The surgical neck is the most common site of fracture, whereas fractures of the anatomic neck are rare.

Articular Head Anatomy

The articular head is spherical, with a diameter of 37 to 57 mm.[8] The inclination and retroversion of the head vary among individuals, as do its medial and posterior offsets. The head is inclined 130° to the shaft and is offset 3 mm posteriorly and 7 mm medially from the center of the shaft. The amount of retroversion can vary from that of the normal, opposite side and ranges from 18° to 40°.[8-10] This range is a result of the variable definition of the humeral neck, which is unlike the femoral neck in that its articular margin varies from the top of the head to the bottom. Varying radiographic techniques and choice of the distal axis also contribute to the degree of normal retroversion. Most studies, however, cite 26° to 31° as average humeral retroversion.[9-12] The large range of normal anatomy has led to the use of the bicipital groove as a guide when restoring the articular anatomy.[13]

Muscular Anatomy

The primary deforming forces in proximal humerus fractures are the pectoralis major and the rotator cuff. The pectoralis major inserts on the shaft below the lesser tuberosity and pulls the shaft anterior and medial (Figure 1). The rotator cuff affects tuberosity displacement and head rotation. The supraspinatus, infraspinatus, and teres minor all insert into individual facets on the greater tuberosity. When fractured, the greater tuberosity can remain intact or fragment into individual facets. The greater tuberosity retracts posteriorly and superiorly by the pull of the supraspina-

FIGURE 1

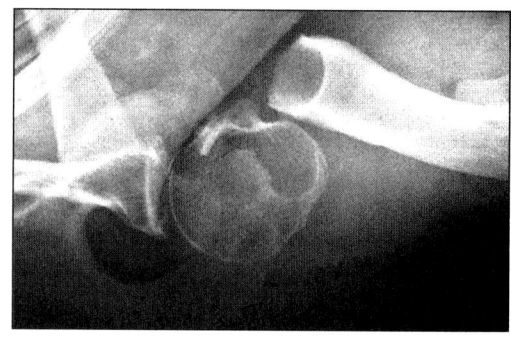

Axillary radiograph of a 63-year-old right-handed man showing anterior shaft displacement in a two-part surgical neck fracture.

tus and infraspinatus. The subscapularis inserts on the lesser tuberosity, and the bicipital groove runs between the two tuberosities. The lesser tuberosity is retracted medially by the pull of the subscapularis. Displacement of the tuberosities is limited by the rotator interval between the supraspinatus and subscapularis. Head displacement is contingent on which structures remain attached to it. For example, a surgical neck fracture in which the greater tuberosity remains attached will have a head that is externally rotated. However, if only the lesser tuberosity remains, the head will be internally rotated. The spinning of the head was termed rotatory subluxation by Neer.

Vascular Anatomy

The proximal humerus receives its blood supply via the distal branches of the axillary artery: the anterior and posterior circumflex humeral arteries. The posterior circumflex humeral artery travels posteriorly with the axillary nerve through the quadrilateral space around the shaft and then anastomoses with the anterior circumflex humeral artery. The anterior circumflex humeral artery arises from the axillary artery at the inferior border of the subscapularis tendon to which it sends a small branch. A small anterolateral branch enters the humeral head to form the arcuate artery, which supplies the humeral head except for a small posterior section. The arcuate artery (of Laing) also receives many small collateral branches from extraosseous vessels. Flow to the humeral head may be compromised by ligation of the arcuate artery distal to these collateral branches.[14] However, complete soft-tissue stripping, in addition to distal ligation, is required to completely halt perfusion of the humeral head in the laboratory setting.[15]

Vascular injuries are infrequent (5% to 6%). The increased incidence of arterial injury in patients with arteriosclerosis may result from decreased vessel wall elasticity.[16] The axillary artery is known as the "tethered trifurcation" at the level of the surgical neck. Most vascular injuries to the arterial supply of the proximal humerus occur at the trifurcation just proximal to the anterior circumflex humeral artery.

Nerve Anatomy

Evaluation of any patient with a proximal humerus fracture must include a complete neurovascular examination because of the close proximity of the axillary nerve and brachial plexus. The brachial plexus (C5-T1) and small contributions from the C3 and C4 roots innervate the shoulder. The axillary nerve travels on the deep surface of the deltoid and wraps around the proximal humerus after entering the quadrilateral space. It then divides into three branches that innervate the teres minor and deltoid. The lateral brachial cutaneous nerve branches off the axillary nerve and travels through the deltoid to the surface to supply sensation over the deltoid. The suprascapular nerve, originating from the upper trunk, innervates the supraspinatus and infraspinatus muscles. The articular branches to the shoulder joint arise from the axillary, suprascapular, and lateral anterior thoracic nerves.

Concurrent injury to the brachial plexus is infrequent (~5%). The axillary nerve is most susceptible to injury in anterior fracture-dislocations because the nerve courses on the inferior capsule and is prone to traction injury or laceration. Electromyographic studies should be completed as a baseline and to monitor for improvement. Exploration for nerve injury should be considered for complete injuries of several months' duration without electromyographic improvement.[17]

Pathomechanics

Fractures of the proximal humerus occur indirectly as a result of rotator cuff traction and humeroglenoid or humeroacromial contact rather than a direct blow to the humerus.[2,18] The most common mechanism of proximal humerus fracture is a fall onto the outstretched arm. Most of these fractures result from falls on level ground in an elderly population in an indoor setting.[2]

High-energy mechanisms, such as a motor vehicle accident or a fall from a height, are more common in a younger population with strong bone. These fractures are usually more severe. Seizures and electrical shock are an indirect mechanism of fracture; with tuberosity fractures seen most commonly after seizures.[19-21]

CLINICAL EVALUATION

Examination

Proximal humerus fractures occur in both young and older populations. A complete history and physical examination must be obtained to determine the mechanism and velocity of fracture and to identify other associated injuries, such as rib, cervical, and scapular fractures, that occur in high-energy trauma.[22] The presentation of proximal humerus fractures is typical; patients will be tender over the shoulder with associated swelling and possible ecchymosis. Ecchymosis, which typically appears within 24 to 48 hours after injury and may extend distally into the arm, forearm, chest wall, and breast over the next 4 to 5 days, is useful in identifying the timing and severity of the injury. Ecchymosis may appear within the first few hours after high-velocity trauma and represents more extensive soft-tissue disruption. The patient will hold the arm in internal rotation. Palpation over the shoulder and any attempted movement of the extremity will elicit pain in the shoulder region. Crepitus can be noted with palpation of the shoulder. Gentle rotation of the humerus and palpation of the fracture can be used as a guide to fracture stability because stable fractures will move as a unit.

A complete neurovascular assessment must be performed because axillary nerve, brachial plexus, and arterial injuries can occur with proximal humerus fractures. Arterial injuries, even in the presence of a normal physical examination, should be suspected in all four-part fracture-dislocations in which the humeral head is in the axilla (Figure 2).

Imaging

Imaging of the shoulder is often difficult and requires careful radiographic views. Careful patient positioning is paramount for diagnosis. The shoulder trauma series consists of a "true" AP scapular view, a lateral "Y" view of the scapula, and an axillary view of the glenohumeral joint

FIGURE 2

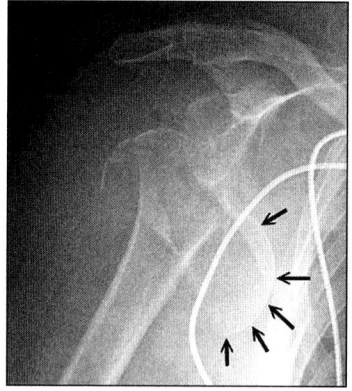

AP radiograph of a 75-year-old right-handed woman with a displaced four-part proximal humerus fracture. Arrows outline the displaced articular surface in the axilla.

FIGURE 3

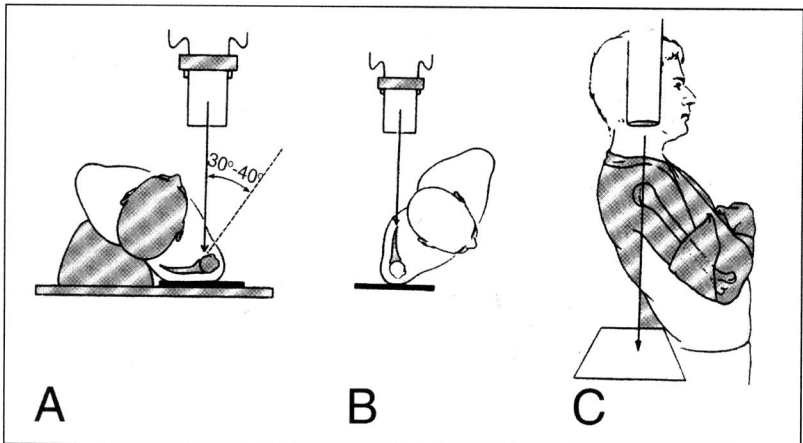

Schematic view of the trauma series. **A**, True scapular AP view; **B**, Scapular lateral view; **C**, Velpeau axillary view. (Reproduced with permission from Levine W, Marra G, Bigliani L (eds): *Fractures of the Shoulder Girdle.* New York, NY, Marcel Dekker, 2003.)

(Figure 3). The abducted axillary view is difficult to obtain and is often painful for the patient. The Velpeau axillary view is preferred in the trauma series. This view is obtained by aiming the x-ray beam down the shoulder from superior to inferior. The patient leans back over the cassette with the arm in a sling. Internal and external rotation AP views of the scapula provide a clear picture of the lesser and greater tuberosities, respectively.

The trauma series, when correctly obtained, provides a clear view of the proximal humerus. CT is helpful in assessing glenoid fractures, posterior dislocations, comminution, and posteriorly displaced greater tuberosity or medially displaced lesser tuberosity fragments that are not well visualized by plain radiographs.

Although rarely indicated in the trauma setting, MRI is used when the patient has symptoms of a preinjury shoulder problem, such as a rotator cuff tear, and in pathologic fracture to evaluate the extent of metastases in the region. MRI also is used to evaluate for nonunion when a patient has persistent pain after the period of fracture healing. No study has supported the routine use of MRI for evaluation of fractures.

CLASSIFICATION

History
The first classification system of humerus fractures was simple: closed versus open in the Edwin Smith Surgical

Papyrus, dating from the seventeenth century BC.[23] In modern times, initial fracture classification focused on the location of the fracture rather than the pattern. In 1896, Kocher,[24] focusing on the location of the fracture, divided proximal humerus fractures into supratubercular, peritubercular, infratubercular, and subtubercular. Codman[25] divided proximal humerus fractures into 11 different types according to the fracture pattern. He described fractures along the lines of the epiphyseal scars, and he observed that fractures occur in several combinations of four parts: the articular surface, humeral shaft, greater tuberosity, and lesser tuberosity (Figure 4). Codman also noted that when loss of all soft-tissue attachments occurred in fracture-dislocations, the head was susceptible to osteonecrosis.

The Watson-Jones[26] system, based on the mechanism of injury, described proximal humerus fractures as impacted adduction, impacted abduction, and a contusion-crack fracture, a fracture of minimal displacement. This system, however, was confusing because the adduction and abduction fracture patterns could be switched if the arm was moved during imaging. Dehne[27] also based his classification system, using the greater tuberosity, shaft, and head, on mechanism of injury. Forced abduction would result in a three-fragment fracture pattern, whereas forced extension resulted in a two-fragment fracture separating the head from the shaft. This was also the mechanism of the head-splitting fracture

FIGURE 4

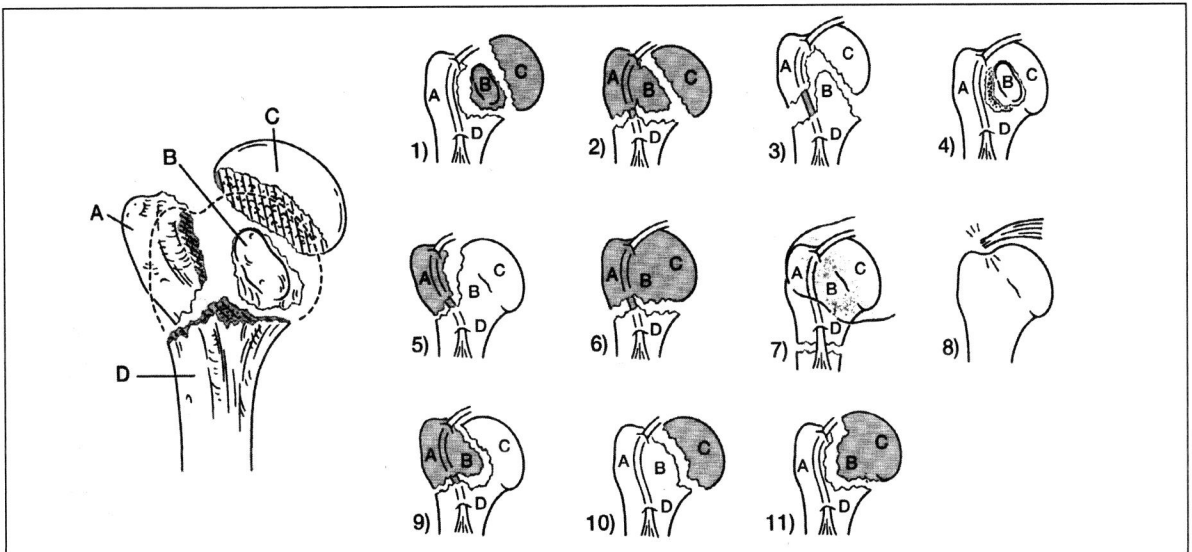

Codman classification of proximal humerus fractures. A = greater tuberosity; B = lesser tuberosity; C = articular surface; D = shaft. (Reproduced with permission from Levine W, Marra G, Bigliani L (eds): *Fractures of the Shoulder Girdle.* New York, NY, Marcel Dekker, 2003.)

in which the head is driven into the glenoid.[27]

The classification system used by De Anquin and De Anquin[28] was similar to the one used by Neer.[29] The proximal humerus was divided into three zones, and impacted and nonimpacted four-fragment fractures were described separately. In the 1960s De Palma and Cautilli[30] distinguished between fracture-dislocations of the glenohumeral joint and rotational deformities in which the head remained in the capsule.

The Neer[29] classification system, published in 1970, is based on displacement of the parts and prognosis determined by head viability. He published results from the observation of 300 randomly selected proximal humerus fractures, focusing on the pattern of displacement rather than the location of the fracture lines. In outcome analysis, he focused on humeral head viability and the glenohumeral relationship.[31]

AO/ASIF Classification System

Jakob and Ganz[32] proposed a classification system based on the study of 730 proximal humerus fractures, which became incorporated into the comprehensive AO system of classifying all long bones. The system emphasizes the vascular supply of the articular portion of the proximal

humerus. The 27 possible subgroups are based on extra-articular or articular involvement, focality, dislocation, and degree of comminution. The vascular supply to the fragment is considered adequate if either tuberosity remains attached to the head.[32,33] This system has not been widely used because of its complexity. It may have a role in clinical research and cohort analysis, but the system's intraobserver and interobserver reliability is similar to that of Neer's system, even among its creators.[34] No long-term results of treatments are based on the AO/ASIF classification system.

Neer Classification System

Fractures are classified by evaluating the displacement of the parts (head, shaft, greater tuberosity, and lesser tuberosity) from each other. To meet the criteria of a part, the fragment must be rotated 45° or 1 cm from another fragment. A proximal humerus with multiple fracture lines may be considered a one-part fracture if there is no significant displacement. A two-part fracture is typically a surgical neck fracture in which the head with attached tuberosities is displaced from the shaft; a displaced greater tuberosity fracture, lesser tuberosity fracture, or anatomic neck fracture is less common. Three-part fractures, which may include head dislocation, involve the surgical neck and one of the tuberosities; the greater tuberosity displaces more commonly than the lesser tuberosity. In four-part fractures, all parts are displaced, and the articular head fragment is devoid of soft-tissue attachments. The exception to this is the valgus-impacted proximal humerus fracture (Figure 5), in which the head is displaced from the glenoid and rotated upward. The head may retain capsular and periosteal attachments along the medial calcar, which might account for the decreased rate of osteonecrosis in this fracture pattern.

The final category is fractures of the articular surface. Articular loss occurs in head-splitting or impaction fractures and fracture-dislocations. These fractures are classified separately in the Neer system because of the poor prognosis for femoral head viability; moreover, fracture-dislocations are delineated based on the anterior or posterior dislocation of the articular fragment. A simplified classification diagram is shown in Figure 6.

Reliability

For effective use, a classification system must have intra- and interobserver reliability and precisely predict prognosis along various treatment algorithms. The Neer system is widely used for classification and treatment of proximal humerus fractures and has been compared to the AO/ASIF classification system.[34-40] Multiple studies report the reliability of the Neer and AO/ASIF systems among both experienced and inexperienced radiologists and orthopaedic surgeons using plain radiographs and radiographs plus CT.

One of the earlier studies by Kristiansen and associates[36] found poor interobserver reliability of the Neer system using AP and lateral radiographs and two pairs of inexperienced observers. The authors concluded that experienced orthopaedic surgeons or radiologists should assess fractures of the proximal humerus.

In other studies, experienced observers and the shoulder trauma series were used to assess the reliability of the Neer and AO/ASIF systems. Siebenrock and Gerber[34] studied radiographs of 95 fractures of the proximal humerus. Five orthopaedic shoulder specialists classified the fractures using the Neer and AO/ASIF systems. They reviewed the radiographs at weeks 0 and 8. The interobserver and intraobserver reliability were found to be fair or poor for both classification systems. Kappa values for interobserver reliability were 0.40 for

FIGURE 5

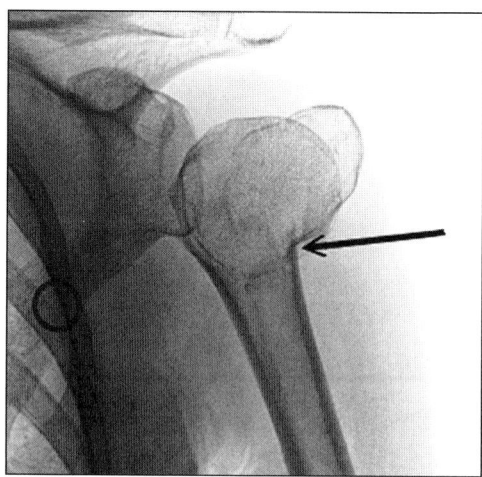

True AP radiograph of the left shoulder in a 59-year-old left-handed woman with a surgical neck fracture in which the head is impacted in a valgus position (arrow). Note the relationship of the greater tuberosity to the humeral shaft: the tuberosity is not truly displaced. The articular surface is in valgus, leaving the greater tuberosity relatively high. Once the articular surface is reduced, the greater tuberosity will be in its anatomic position.

the Neer system and 0.53 for the AO/ASIF system. Reliability for the AO/ASIF classification declined when the fractures were subclassified (kappa values: groups, 0.60; subgroups, 0.58). The addition of a third radiograph to complete the trauma series significantly improved the reliability values of both classifications compared with values obtained with only two perpendicular projections. The authors concluded that neither the Neer nor the AO/ASIF classification of proximal humerus fractures is sufficiently reproducible to allow meaningful comparison of similarly classified fractures in different studies.[34]

Sidor and associates[38] found similar results using trauma series radiographs of 50 fractures to assess the intra- and interobserver reliability of the simplified Neer classification system, which has been reduced from 16 categories to 6 more general categories based on fracture type. An orthopaedic shoulder specialist, an orthopaedic traumatologist, a skeletal radiologist, and two orthopaedic residents reviewed the radiographs 6 months apart. All five observers agreed on the final classification for 32% and 30% of the fractures on the first and second viewings, respectively. Paired comparisons

FIGURE 6

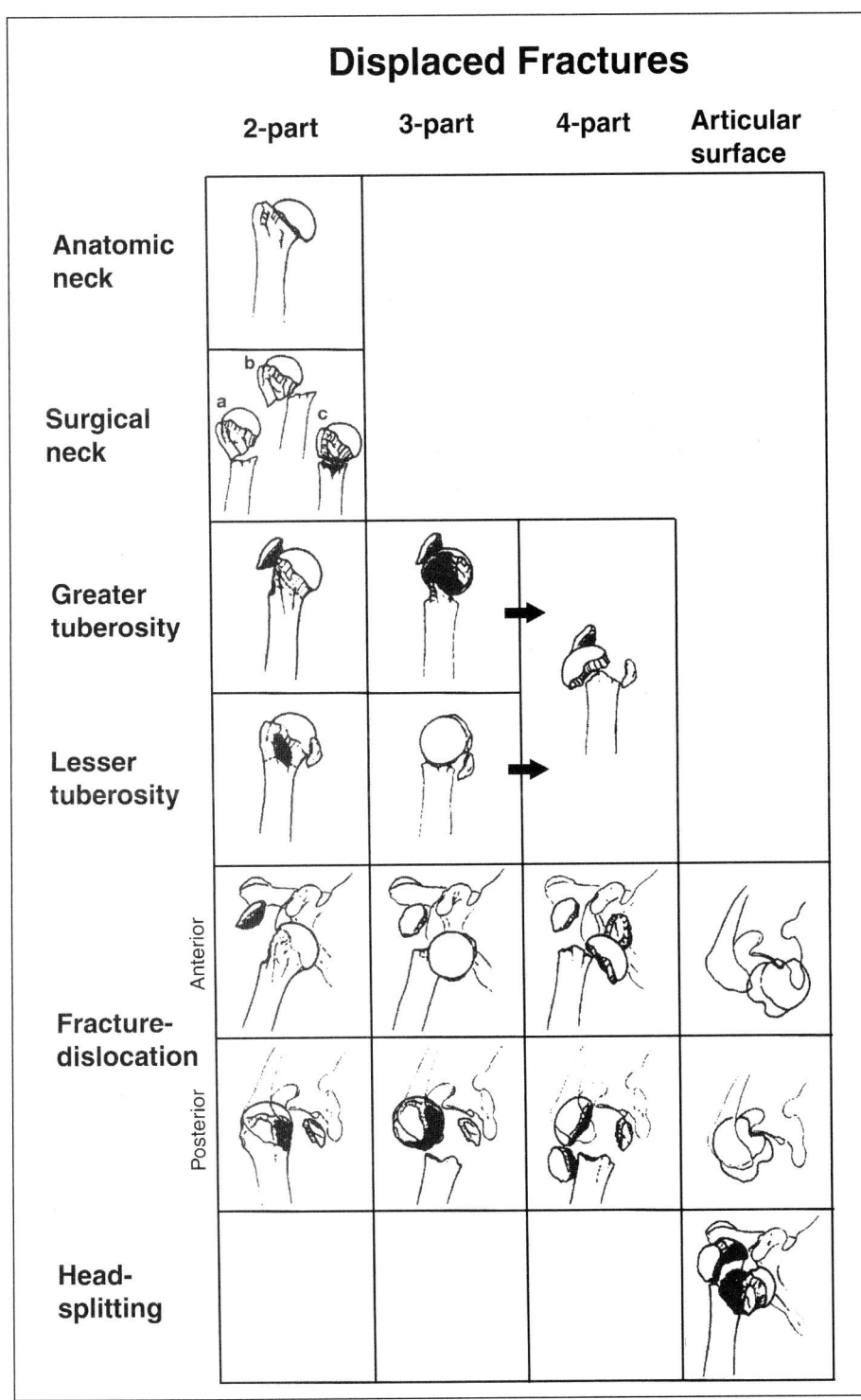

The Neer classification system. (Reproduced with permission from Levine W, Marra G, Bigliani L (eds): *Fractures of the Shoulder Girdle.* New York, NY, Marcel Dekker, 2003.)

between the five observers showed a mean reliability coefficient of 0.48 (range, 0.43 to 0.58) for the first viewing and 0.52 (range, 0.37 to 0.62) for the second viewing. The authors concluded that even the simplification of the Neer classification system did not significantly improve either inter- or intraobserver reliability.[38]

The Neer classification system also has been evaluated for reliability when CT scans augment plain radiography. Sjoden and associates[39] assessed the reliability of the Neer and AO/ASIF fracture classification systems using 26 proximal humerus fractures that were independently classified by five radiologists and five orthopaedic surgeons viewing plain radiographs and CT scans. The authors found that there was moderate agreement using the Neer classification, but only fair agreement with the AO/ASIF classification. The kappa values were 0.42 and 0.31, respectively, in the first assessment and 0.45 and 0.30, respectively, in the second assessment. Intraobserver reliability ranged from slight to almost perfect agreement with the Neer system (kappa range, 0.20 to 0.85) and slight to moderate agreement with AO/ASIF (kappa range, 0.16 to 0.60). They concluded that even with CT scans, the Neer and AO/ASIF fracture classifications have a low reliability, and neither system is reliable enough to allow comparisons of different studies.[39]

Bernstein and associates[35] assessed the Neer classification system on the basis of the plain radiographs and CT scans of 20 fractures of the proximal humerus. Two fifth-year orthopaedic residents and two fellowship-trained shoulder surgeons were asked to classify the fractures according to the Neer system and a modified system (in which fracture lines were considered but displacement was not) and asked to recommend treatment for the fracture. Intraobserver reliability was moderate (0.64) with plain radiographs, slightly improved (0.72) with the addition of CT scans, and very little difference in the modified system (0.68). Reliability in treatment recommendations was strong (0.84). The mean kappa coefficients for interobserver reliability were 0.52, 0.50, 0.56, and 0.65, respectively. The authors concluded that the classification of shoulder fractures remains difficult because even experts cannot uniformly agree which fragments are fractured, and they believed that optimum patient care might require the development of new imaging modalities and not necessarily new classification systems.[35]

Bernstein and associates'[35] study results agree with those of Sallay and associates,[37] who also augmented plain radiography with CT in the assessment of reliability. These authors concluded that the addition of three-dimensional CT scans did not improve the reliability and that poor agreement for the purpose of classification seems to occur at the description of the fracture.[37]

The Neer classification system is widely used by orthopaedic surgeons for the diagnosis and treatment of proximal humerus fractures. Its success is based on its anatomic consideration of soft-tissue attachments and emphasis on the degree of displacement rather than the fracture pattern. Imaging of the shoulder is a complex and difficult task. Fracture fragmentation is not always well visualized on CT scans and plain radiographs, causing the classification system to lose reliability. Often, only surgical exploration can accurately determine the fracture pattern. Despite these concerns, the Neer system has evolved and provides the surgeon with a logical rationale for management and surgical planning based on known anatomy and proximal humerus fracture patterns.

TREATMENT

Most proximal humerus fractures can be successfully treated nonsurgically because they are not sufficiently displaced or angulated to require surgical intervention. The two-part nondisplaced proximal humerus fracture is the most common variation,[30,41] and three- and four-part fractures represent 13% to 16% of all proximal humerus fractures.[1] Approximately 20% of fractures require surgical intervention.[30] Nondisplaced or minimally displaced proximal humerus fractures do well with nonsurgical management; however, the treatment of comminuted displaced fractures is controversial.[41,42]

The gold standard outcome of any fracture treatment is a pain-free extremity with full range of motion. In Neer's classic study of proximal humerus fractures, more than 1 cm of displacement or 45° of angulation was considered an indication for surgical management. In practice, a good outcome does not always require a near-anatomic reduction. As long as there is solid bony contact and a vascular supply, angulation is well compensated for by shoulder motion. In general, considerations in determining treatment for a fracture must

FIGURE 7

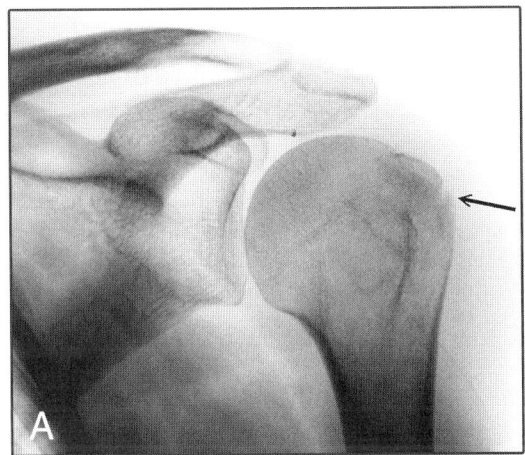

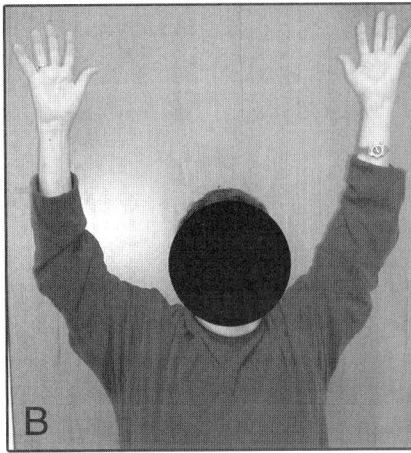

A, True AP radiograph of a 56-year-old left-handed woman with a nondisplaced greater tuberosity fracture (arrow). **B,** Clinical photograph 3 months following fracture. Physical therapy was instituted 14 days after the fracture occurred.

include an assessment of the fracture pattern, bone quality, status of the rotator cuff, and the patient's age, activity level, and preinjury health. A patient with low demands or medical contraindications to surgical intervention will be served best with nonsurgical management. A patient with dementia or inability to participate in rehabilitation also should be managed nonsurgically.

Minimally Displaced Fractures

Almost all minimally displaced fractures of the proximal humerus are managed nonsurgically. The rare indications for surgical management of these fractures include ipsilateral neurovascular injury requiring exploration, open fracture, or polytrauma.

The principles for nonsurgical management for nondisplaced or minimally displaced fractures are early protection combined with gradual mobilization. This treatment entails sling immobilization for the first 7 to 10 days. A swathe can be used for comfort the first few days, but many patients find it difficult to manage and uncomfortable after 2 to 3 days of use. The patient is instructed in and encouraged to begin finger, hand, wrist, and elbow motion immediately. By 2 weeks, formal physical therapy may begin with gentle active-assisted range-of-motion exercises. By 6 weeks, light resistive exercises may begin.

Koval and associates[43] studied functional outcome of minimally displaced proximal humerus fractures; 104 patients with a one-part fracture were managed with a standardized physical therapy regimen and followed for more than 1 year. Clinical outcome, after an average of 41 months, was assessed on the basis of pain, function, and shoulder range of motion. All fractures went on to bony union, functional recovery averaged 94%, and 46% of patients had 100% functional recovery. The percentage of good and excellent results was significantly greater ($P < 0.01$), and motion was significantly better ($P < 0.01$) in patients who began formal physical therapy within 14 days of injury.

Tuberosity Fractures

Historically, greater tuberosity fractures were well described by Taylor[44] in 1908. Abduction traction, casting, or bracing was used to bring the humeral head to the superiorly displaced greater tuberosity.[45,46] The amount of tuberosity displacement is the primary consideration in determining whether surgical or nonsurgical treatment is indicated. Most nondisplaced and minimally displaced tuberosity fractures can be treated nonsurgically (Figure 7); most displaced fractures require surgical treatment. As always, the patient's age, lifestyle, and preinjury level of function are important in the decision-making process. In greater tuberosity fracture-dislocations, the greater tuberosity will often become nondisplaced following reduction.

Impingement may occur when the greater tuberosity is displaced more than 5 mm. External rotation will be limited with posterior greater tuberosity displacement of more than 10 mm. In sedentary patients, slightly more displacement may be tolerated without functional loss. Therefore, nonsurgical treatment of greater tuberosity fractures is limited to those patients with nondisplaced or minimally displaced fractures, low-demand patients, and patients unable to follow rehabilitation instructions. Nonsurgical management consists of a brief period of immobilization followed by formal physical therapy to restore motion.

An isolated lesser tuberosity fracture without an associated posterior dislocation or surgical neck fracture is extremely rare. The lesser tuberosity fragment displaces medially secondary to the pull of the subscapularis, and a large fragment will impede internal rotation. Recommendations for surgical management include a fracture of the lesser tuberosity with large fragments or a fracture containing articular surface. In select patients, nonsurgical management is possible with early mobilization and therapy.[47]

Surgical Neck Fractures

Surgical neck fractures comprise 60% to 65% of all adult proximal humerus fractures. Almost 80% of these fractures are minimally displaced and amenable to nonsurgical management. Indications for surgical management include displacement, polytrauma, association with other upper extremity fractures, vascular injury, and open fracture.

If, on first evaluation, the fracture is displaced but not impacted, closed reduction may be attempted at the time of injury. After sedation or a hematoma block, the arm is adducted and flexed 90° to relax the pectoralis, and a posterolateral translation force is applied with longitudinal traction. Once reduced, the fracture can be impacted for stability. If closed reduction is successful and the fracture is stable, then the fracture can be treated as minimally displaced; however, it requires close monitoring until union is achieved. Two-part fracture-dislocations can be treated nonsurgically if the fragments are not displaced or are minimally displaced following glenohumeral reduction.

The amount of displacement is critical in deciding between surgical and nonsurgical management. Malunion can be tolerated if the relationship between the articular surface and tuberosity is intact. In the elderly or the low-demand patient, bony contact may be all that is necessary to create a functional malunion. In active individuals, less than 50% shaft diameter displacement and less than 45° angulation in the dominant arm is well tolerated. Fractures angulated in varus or valgus, comminuted fractures, and completely displaced surgical neck fractures have poor results with nonsurgical treatment because they are unstable and will redisplace after reduction. Chun and associates,[47] reviewing 56 surgical neck fractures that were treated nonsurgically, found that only 55% (31 patients) had an excellent or good result at an average of 6.6 years. Motion also was limited, with a mean forward elevation of 104°.

In an earlier study, Clifford[48] reported 15% poor or unsatisfactory results in 80 proximal humerus fractures 18 months after injury. The severity of the fracture, duration of immobilization, and duration of therapy all independently affected the result. Patients with minimally displaced fractures had better results (94% satisfactory) with nonsurgical management than patients with displaced fractures (68% satisfactory).[48]

Management of surgical neck fractures depends largely on the bone quality, functional demand, and cognitive ability of the patient. Closed reduction and nonsurgical management is best reserved for minimally to less than 50% displaced fractures in patients who can be mobilized quickly and participate in rehabilitation. Displaced fractures and active patients have better results with surgical management.

Three-Part Fractures

The three-part fracture has fracture lines that occur through the surgical neck and tuberosities. The degree of displacement of the parts depends largely on the proximity of the fracture line to the rotator cuff because the muscle provides the deforming forces. These fractures are unstable because of opposing muscles and associated soft-tissue destruction around the fracture.

Treatment options include closed reduction and management, closed reduction and percutaneous fixation, and open reduction and internal fixation (ORIF). Nonsurgical management of three-part fractures follows the same principles as management of minimally displaced fractures. Closed reduction is attempted but is often unsuccessful because of the degree of displacement and rotatory subluxation of the head. Attempts at closed reduction should be minimal because further fragmentation and bony destruction can occur. The shoulder is immobilized for 7 to 10 days with a sling, and formal rehabilitation is begun as soon as the patient can tolerate motion.

Most three-part fractures are treated surgically in the absence of medical contraindications because of the deformity of the proximal humerus. However, several studies have reviewed the results of nonsurgical treatment of three-part fractures and found that a good functional outcome can be achieved.[49-51]

Lill and associates[49] evaluated patients with displaced (angulation of the humeral head > 45° and/or shaft displacement > 1 cm and displacement of the greater tuberosity > 0.5 cm) proximal humerus fractures treated nonsurgically and retrospectively followed for an average of 20 months after injury. Twenty-three patients had excellent or good results, and seven patients had moderate or poor results. Poor results resulted primarily from persistent pain in range of motion and loss of strength. Radiographic assessment revealed 23 patients with persistent axial deviation, 14 patients with arthrosis, and 8 patients with humeral head necrosis. They concluded that four-part fractures had poor results and should be treated surgically but that two- and three-part fractures can be treated nonsurgically and have a good outcome.[49]

In another long-term study, Zyto[50] retrospectively reviewed the clinical and radiographic results of nonsurgical treatment in 17 patients with displaced multifragmented fractures of the proximal humerus with a minimum follow-up of 10 years. The review found low Constant scores in the three- and four-part fracture groups (59 and 47, respectively), although only four patients had mild pain, and all had satisfactory range of motion. Radiographic examination revealed severe osteoarthritis in one shoulder and humeral head osteonecrosis in two shoulders. The authors concluded that nonsurgical management of three-part fractures should be considered because most patients were content with their shoulder function 10 years after injury.[50]

In a prospective study, Zyto and associates[51] randomized 40 patients (mean age, 74 years) with displaced three- or four-part fractures of the humerus to either nonsurgical treatment or tension-band osteosynthesis. Clinical follow-up at 1 year and again at 3 to 5 years showed no functional differences between the two groups. Radiologic review showed that although surgery had improved the position of the fractured humeral head, this improvement was not reflected in improved function. The authors concluded that tension-band wiring in the elderly did not improve the functional outcome compared with nonsurgical treatment.[51]

Four-Part Fractures

Four-part fractures, with the exception of valgus-impacted head fractures, leave the articular segment without vascular supply. Treatment options include closed management, ORIF, and humeral head replacement. Most of these fractures or fracture-dislocations are treated surgically as a result of the poor functional outcome of nonsurgical treatment.[49,52] Nonsurgical treatment for four-part fractures results in a high incidence of complications, including osteonecrosis, mal-union, nonunion, and posttraumatic osteoarthritis.[52] If nonsurgical management is elected, the principles of treatment are the same as for other proximal humerus fractures. Closed reduction is attempted, the patient is immobilized for a short period of time with a sling, and formal physical therapy is begun 2 weeks after injury when the fracture has become more stable.

Fracture-Dislocations and Articular Fractures

Three- and four-part fracture-dislocations require surgical treatment. These fractures are associated with an increased incidence of myositis ossificans with repeated attempts at closed reduction or with delayed ORIF. Articular surface fractures are most often associated with posterior dislocations and require ORIF or hemiarthroplasty. Closed management should be considered only if there are severe medical contraindications to surgery.

CONCLUSIONS

Proximal humerus fractures are common, especially in the elderly, and most can be treated nonsurgically with excellent functional recovery. Classification systems provide an algorithm for diagnosis, treatment, and prognosis. The Neer classification system is successful because it is based on the regional anatomy of the proximal humerus and places great importance on the deforming forces of the shoulder. Evaluation of proximal humerus fractures requires an understanding of the complex anatomy, especially the deforming forces.

Review of the literature demonstrates that minimally displaced fractures are successfully treated nonsurgically, and a better functional outcome is achieved if formal rehabilitation is begun within 14 days of injury. Two- and three-part fractures also do well with nonsurgical treatment if the treatment decision is based on patient characteristics, specifically preinjury function, health, bone quality, and the fracture pattern. Four-part fractures, because of the long-term poor functional results of painful malunion or nonunion, are best treated with surgical intervention.

REFERENCES

1. Horak J, Nilsson BE: Epidemiology of fracture of the upper end of the humerus. *Clin Orthop* 1975;112:250-253.
2. Lind T, Kroner K, Jensen J: The epidemiology of fractures of the proximal humerus. *Arch Orthop Trauma Surg* 1989;108:285-287.
3. Kannus P, Palvanen M, Niemi S, Parkkari J, Jarvinen M, Vuori I: Osteoporotic fractures of the proximal humerus in elderly Finnish persons: Sharp increase in 1970-1998 and alarming projections for the new millennium. *Acta Orthop Scand* 2000;71:465-470.
4. Nordqvist A, Petersson CJ: Incidence and causes of shoulder girdle injuries in an urban population. *J Shoulder Elbow Surg* 1995;4:107-112.
5. Kelsey JL, Browner WS, Seeley DG, Nevitt MC, Cummings SR: Risk factors for fractures of the distal forearm and proximal humerus: The Study of Osteoporotic Fractures Research Group. *Am J Epidemiol* 1992;135:477-489.
6. Lee SH, Dargent-Molina P, Breart G: Risk factors for fractures of the proximal humerus: Results from the EPIDOS prospective study. *J Bone Miner Res* 2002;17:817-825.
7. Naranja RJ Jr, Iannotti JP: Displaced three- and four-part proximal humerus fractures: Evaluation and management. *J Am Acad Orthop Surg* 2000;8:373-382.
8. Boileau P, Walch G: The three-dimensional geometry of the proximal humerus: Implications for surgical technique and prosthetic design. *J Bone Joint Surg Br* 1997;79:857-865.
9. Debevoise NT, Hyatt GW, Townsend GB: Humeral torsion in recurrent shoulder dislocations: A technic of determination by x-ray. *Clin Orthop* 1971;76:87-93.
10. Hill JA, Tkach L, Hendrix RW: A study of glenohumeral orientation in patients with anterior recurrent shoulder dislocations using computerized axial tomography. *Orthop Rev* 1989;18:84-91.
11. Krahl VE: The phylogeny and ontogeny of humeral torsion. *Am J Phys Anthropol* 1976;45:595-599.
12. Kronberg M, Brostrom LA, Soderlund V: Retroversion of the humeral head in the normal shoulder and its relationship to the normal range of motion. *Clin Orthop* 1990;253:113-117.
13. Tillet E, Smit M, Fulcher M: Anatomic determination of humeral head retroversion: The relationship of the central axis of the humeral head to the bicipital groove. *J Shoulder Elbow Surg* 1993;2:255-256.
14. Gerber C, Hersche O, Berberat C: The clinical relevance of posttraumatic avascular necrosis of the humeral head. *J Shoulder Elbow Surg* 1998;7:586-590.
15. Brooks CH, Revell WJ, Heatley FW: Vascularity of the humeral head after proximal humeral fractures: An anatomical cadaver study. *J Bone Joint Surg Br* 1993;75:132-136.
16. Manak P, Klein J: Axillary artery injury in closed fracture of the humeral neck. *Acta Univ Palacki Olomuc Fac Med* 1996;140:87-88.
17. Visser CP, Coene LN, Brand R, Tavy DL: Nerve lesions in proximal humeral fractures. *J Shoulder Elbow Surg* 2001;10:421-427.
18. Gold AM: Fractured neck of the humerus with separation and dislocation of the humeral head (Fracture-dislocation of the shoulder, severe type). *Bull Hosp Joint Dis* 1971;32:87-99.
19. Salem MI: Bilateral anterior fracture-dislocation of the shoulder joints due to severe electric shock. *Injury* 1983;14:361-363.
20. Desai KB, Ribbans WJ, Taylor GJ: Incidence of five common fracture types in an institutional epileptic population. *Injury* 1996;27:97-100.
21. Green A, Izzi J Jr: Isolated fractures of the greater tuberosity of the proximal humerus. *J Shoulder Elbow Surg* 2003;12:641-649.
22. Rose SH, Melton LJ III, Morrey BF, Ilstrup DM, Riggs BL: Epidemiologic features of humeral fractures. *Clin Orthop* 1982;168:24-30.
23. Breasted J: *The Edwin Smith Surgical Papyrus.* Chicago, IL, University of Chicago Press, 1930, p 596.
24. Kocher T: *Beiträge zur Kenntnis einiger Praktisch Wichtiger Frakurformen.* Basel, Switzerland, Carl Sallmann, 1896.

25. Codman E: Rupture of the supraspinatus tendon and other lesions in or about the subacromial bursa, in Codman E (ed): *The Shoulder*. Boston, MA, Thomas Todd, 1934.

26. Watson-Jones R: Fracture of the neck of the humerus, in *Fractures and Other Bone and Joint Injuries*. Baltimore, MD, Williams and Wilkins, 1940, pp 289-297.

27. Dehne E: Fractures of the upper end of the humerus. *Surg Clin N Am* 1945;25:28-47.

28. De Anquin C, De Anquin C: Prosthetic replacement in the treatment of serious fractures of the proximal humerus, in *Shoulder Surgery*. Berlin, Germany, Springer-Verlag, 1982, pp 207-217.

29. Neer CS II: Displaced proximal humeral fractures: I. Classification and evaluation. *J Bone Joint Surg Am* 1970;52:1077-1089.

30. De Palma A, Cautilli R: Fractures of the upper end of the humerus. *Clin Orthop* 1961;20:73-93.

31. Neer CT, Brown T, McLaughlin H: Fracture of the neck of the humerus with dislocation of the head fragment. *Am J Surg* 1953;85:252-258.

32. Jakob RP, Ganz R: Proximal humerus fractures. *Helv Chir Acta* 1982;48:595-610.

33. Müller M, Nazarian S, Koch P: *The Comprehensive Classification of Fractures of the Long Bones*. Berlin, Germany, Springer-Verlag, 1990.

34. Siebenrock KA, Gerber C: The reproducibility of classification of fractures of the proximal end of the humerus. *J Bone Joint Surg Am* 1993;75:1751-1755.

35. Bernstein J, Adler LM, Blank JE, Dalsey RM, Williams GR, Iannotti JP: Evaluation of the Neer system of classification of proximal humeral fractures with computerized tomographic scans and plain radiographs. *J Bone Joint Surg Am* 1996;78:1371-1375.

36. Kristiansen B, Andersen UL, Olsen CA, Varmarken JE: The Neer classification of fractures of the proximal humerus: An assessment of interobserver variation. *Skeletal Radiol* 1988;17:420-422.

37. Sallay PI, Pedowitz RA, Mallon WJ, Vandemark RM, Dalton JD, Speer KP: Reliability and reproducibility of radio-graphic interpretation of proximal humeral fracture pathoanatomy. *J Shoulder Elbow Surg* 1997;6:60-69.

38. Sidor ML, Zuckerman JD, Lyon T, Koval K, Cuomo F, Schoenberg N: The Neer classification system for proximal humeral fractures: An assessment of interobserver reliability and intraobserver reproducibility. *J Bone Joint Surg Am* 1993;75:1745-1750.

39. Sjoden GO, Movin T, Guntner P, et al: Poor reproducibility of classification of proximal humeral fractures: Additional CT of minor value. *Acta Orthop Scand* 1997;68:239-242.

40. Soderlund V, Kronberg M, Brostrom LA: Radiologic assessment of humeral head retroversion: Description of a new method *Acta Radiol* 1989;30:501-505.

41. Mills HJ, Horne G: Fractures of the proximal humerus in adults. *J Trauma* 1985;25:801-805.

42. Cofield RH: Comminuted fractures of the proximal humerus. *Clin Orthop* 1988;230:49-57.

43. Koval KJ, Gallagher MA, Marsicano JG, Cuomo F, McShinawy A, Zuckerman JD: Functional outcome after minimally displaced fractures of the proximal part of the humerus. *J Bone Joint Surg Am* 1997;79:203-207.

44. Taylor H: Isolated fracture of the greater tuberosity of the humerus. *Ann Surg* 1908;54:10-12.

45. Miller S: Practical points in the diagnosis and treatment of fractures of the upper fourth of the humerus. *Indust Med* 1940;9:458-460.

46. Sever J: Fracture of the head of the humerus: Treatment and results. *N Engl J Med* 1937;216:1100-1107.

47. Chun J, Groh G, Rockwood CA: Two-part fractures of the proximal humerus. *J Shoulder Elbow Surg* 1994;3:273-287.

48. Clifford PC: Fractures of the neck of the humerus: A review of the late results. *Injury* 1980;11:91-95.

49. Lill H, Bewer A, Korner J, et al: Conservative treatment of dislocated proximal humeral fractures. *Zentralbl Chir* 2001;126:205-210.

50. Zyto K: Non-operative treatment of comminuted fractures of the proximal humerus in elderly patients. *Injury* 1998;29:349-352.

51. Zyto K, Ahrengart L, Sperber A, Tornkvist H: Treatment of displaced proximal humeral fractures in elderly patients. *J Bone Joint Surg Br* 1997;79:412-417.

52. Stableforth PG: Four-part fractures of the neck of the humerus. *J Bone Joint Surg Br* 1984;66:104-108.

CHAPTER 2

PERCUTANEOUS TREATMENT OF PROXIMAL HUMERUS FRACTURES

PETER J. MILLET, MD, MSc
JON J.P. WARNER, MD

Proximal humerus fractures are common, and about 80% are well managed nonsurgically. The remaining 20% present a therapeutic challenge because surgical stabilization is necessary to ensure healing and to optimize function. The priorities in surgical stabilization of proximal humerus fractures are (1) restoring the anatomic relationship between the tuberosities and the articular head fragment and (2) maintaining vascularity of the articular fragment.[1] Open reduction and internal fixation may allow for rigid fracture fixation, but soft-tissue dissection may endanger residual vascularity of the articular segment. Closed reduction followed by percutaneous fixation reduces risk from soft-tissue dissection and may reduce the fracture indirectly, achieving provisional fixation for anatomic healing. This technique requires meticulous attention to detail and teamwork among the surgeon, surgical assistants, nursing staff, and anesthesia staff.

HISTORY

Closed reduction and percutaneous fixation was first described by Bohler[2] for the treatment of pediatric proximal humerus fractures. He reduced the fracture with the patient under general anesthesia and provisionally fixed the humeral head fragment to the shaft using percutaneously placed pins. This method then was adapted to the treatment of fractures in adults. Initially, the technique was applied to the management of two-part surgical neck fractures[3] where it was as successful as open methods. More recently, closed reduction and percutaneous fixation with pins and cannulated screws has been applied to the management of three- and even four-part proximal humerus fractures.[4-6] Although these approaches to more complex fractures are challenging, vascularity of the humeral head seems to be more reliably preserved than in open treatments that require soft-tissue dissection to place rigid fixation implants.[7] The incidence of osteonecrosis is reduced with these methods[4-6,8-12] because the prinicipal vascular supply to the humeral head, the ascending branch of the anterior circumflex humeral artery, is left undisturbed with no dissection in the region of the bicipital groove or around the subscapularis (Figure 1). Indeed, this method has been termed "bio-logical" fixation.[1] The learning curve clearly is steeper for three- and four-part fractures than for two-part surgical neck fractures.

INDICATIONS

The specific indications for closed reduction and percutaneous pinning include proximal humerus fractures without significant comminution in patients with good quality bone who are willing to comply with the postoperative care plan, which includes serial radiographs

FIGURE 1

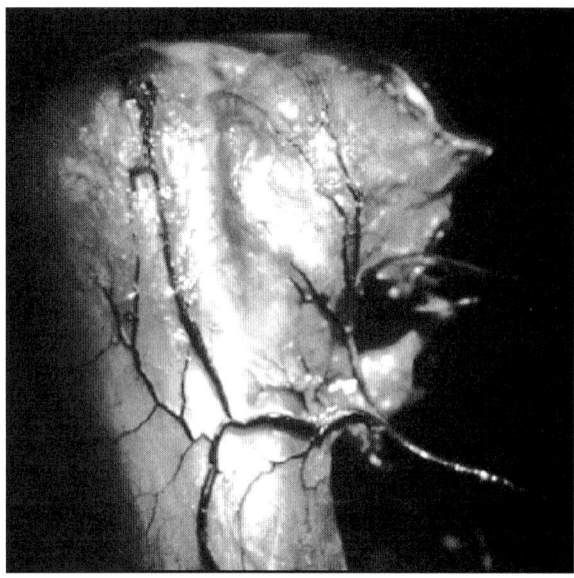

Articular vascularization of the humeral head. *(Reproduced with permission from Gerber C, Schneeberger AG, Vinh TS: The arterial vascularization of the humeral head: An anatomical study.* J Bone Joint Surg Am *1990;72:1486-1494.)*

and shoulder immobilization for 4 to 6 weeks. Certain fracture patterns are easier to manage than others, and these are outlined briefly below.

Two-Part Surgical Neck Fractures: The Shallow Learning Curve

The ideal indication for closed reduction and percutaneous pinning is a two-part surgical neck fracture in which there is marked displacement and/or angulation that will not achieve acceptable healing and restore function (Figure 2). Most patients with these fractures are younger and have good quality bone that permits secure fixation once reduction is accomplished. Patient compliance with postoperative care also is very important.

Three-Part Valgus-Impacted Fractures: The Steeper Learning Curve

This distinct fracture pattern recently has been recognized as being amenable to closed reduction and percutaneous fixation. It is more difficult to treat than the two-part fracture pattern because it requires manipulation of the articular segment into its proper position followed by stable fixation of the tuberosity to the head and to the shaft (Figure 3).

FIGURE 2

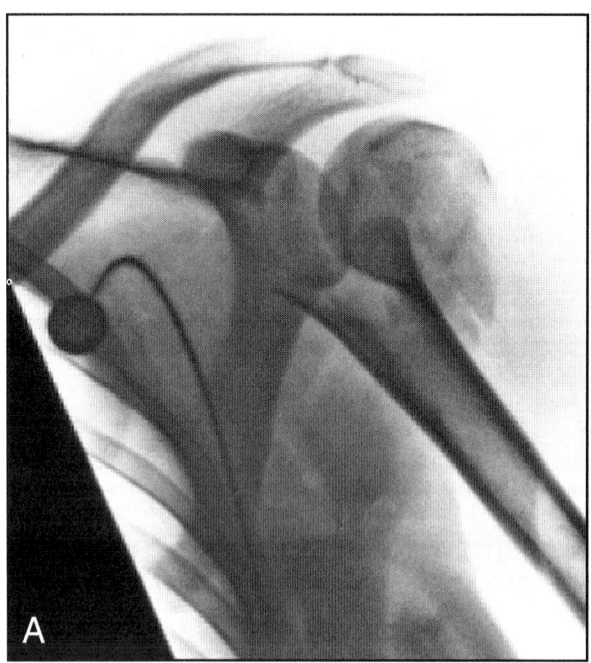

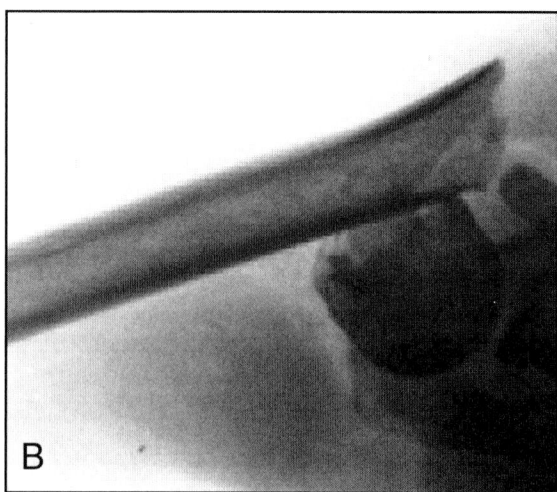

AP **(A)** and axillary **(B)** radiographs showing a two-part surgical neck fracture with complete anterior displacement of the shaft. *(Courtesy of Christian Gerber, MD).*

FIGURE 3

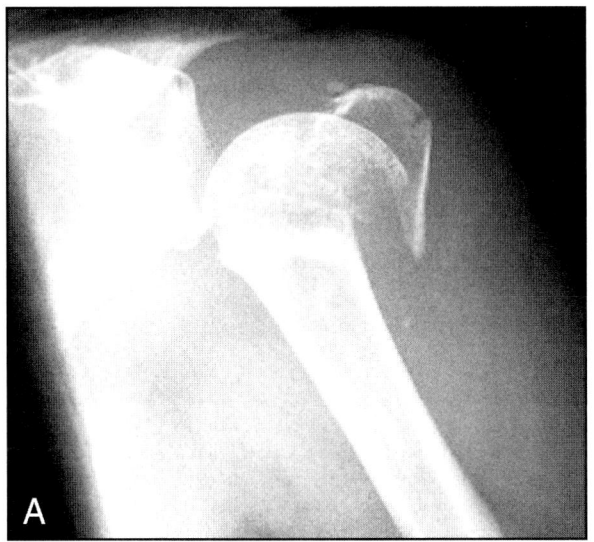 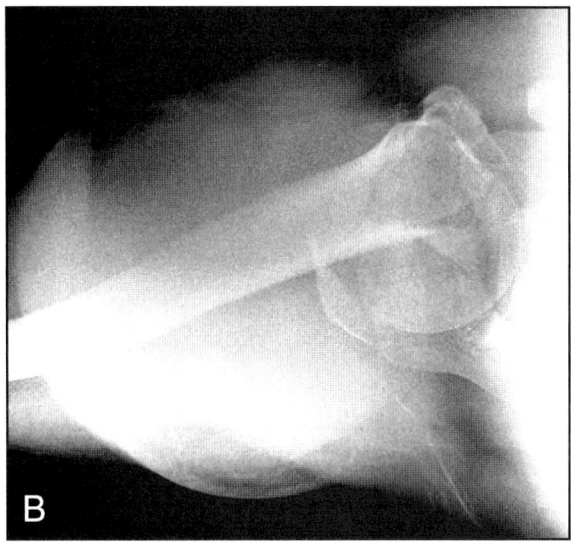

AP **(A)** and axillary **(B)** radiographs of a three-part valgus-impacted fracture.

Four-Part Fractures: The Steepest Learning Curve

Four-part fracture configurations are challenging because adequate reduction and fixation require manipulation of tuberosity fragments into position with percutaneous hooks and pins, followed by stable fixation using combinations of pins and screws (Figure 4).

CONTRAINDICATIONS

Severe comminution and osteopenia are absolute contraindications to closed reduction and percutaneous fixation (Figure 5). Inability to reduce fracture fragments is another reason to abandon this approach and convert to open reduction. Fracture-dislocations also may be impossible to manage using a closed technique. Finally, patients who will not be compliant with postoperative immobilization and the need for pin removal are not good candidates for this method of treatment.

SURGICAL TECHNIQUE

The first and perhaps most important step in achieving a good outcome is proper patient selection. This decision-making step is essential, and guidelines have been outlined in the previous sections. The next key steps are technical and include careful planning and preparation so that all of the appropriate equipment and the necessary team are available. The proper operating room setup is essential, and nursing and anesthesia staff should be aware of the specific positioning needs. The fluoroscopic C-arm operator should rehearse the steps needed to obtain proper, repeatable, biplanar radiographs before the patient's arm is prepared and draped so that the C-arm can be positioned easily and without error during the procedure. Finally, an assistant should be present who understands how to achieve and maintain the reduction and then allow for fixation.

Access to the fractured shoulder is paramount. Specific instrument requirements include a beach chair that allows for complete access to the shoulder for fluoroscopic imaging or a long beanbag that can be contoured to support the patient and allow access to the shoulder. A mechanical arm holder can also help significantly. Reduction instruments should include bone elevators and hooks to manipulate fragments. The necessary implants are 2.5-mm terminally threaded pins (terminal threads reduce chance of migration out of bone) and 4.0-mm cannulated screws. Finally, a drill with a quick-release for the pins and the appropriate chuck attachment for the cannulated screws should be available.

FIGURE 4

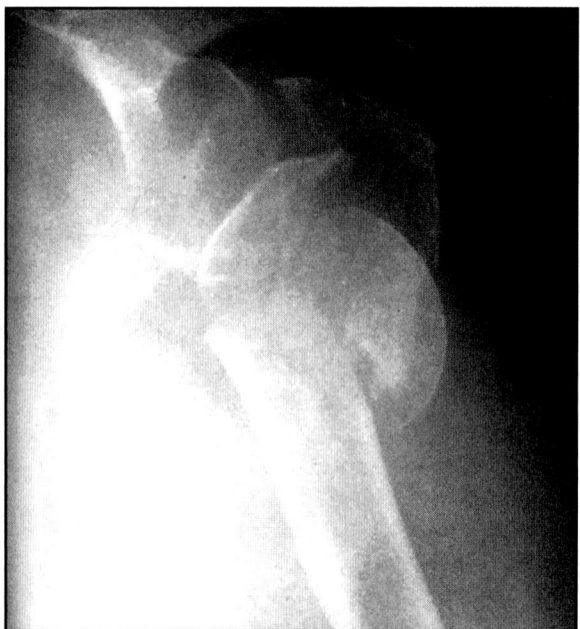

Four-part fracture *(Courtesy of Evan Flatow, MD)*

FIGURE 5

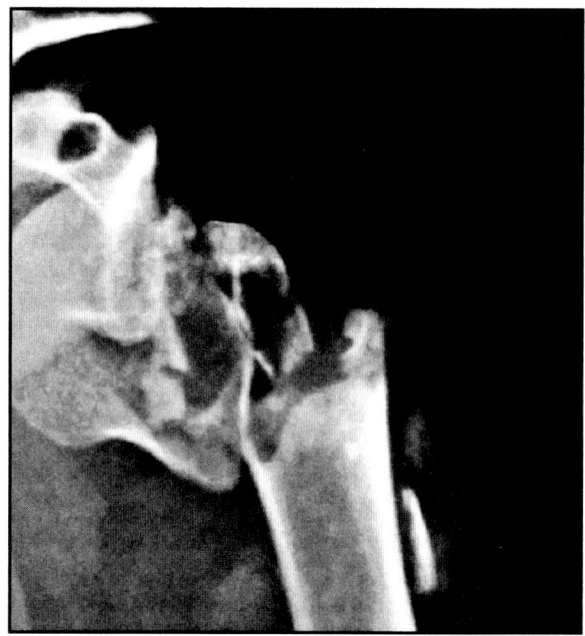

Severe metaphyseal-diaphyseal comminution in a patient with an anterior dislocation. This fracture is not amenable to closed reduction and percutaneous fixation. *(Courtesy of Christian Gerber, MD)*

Positioning

The patient is positioned on a special beach chair or on a regular operating room table with a long bean-bag contoured medial to the scapula to ensure that the entire shoulder girdle is freely exposed for fluoroscopic imaging (Figure 6). A fluoroscopic C-arm is then oriented parallel to the table so that it comes either over or under the shoulder from a position at the head of the table (Figure 7). It may be necessary, depending on the size of the room, to angle the table and move it downward in the room to make space for the C-arm. The image receiver is positioned on the opposite side of the table toward the foot so that the surgeon can see it easily while performing the reduction and fixation. The C-arm is then rotated into an AP view and an axillary view to ensure these views can be obtained easily once the patient's shoulder is prepared and draped.

Closed Reduction

The patient's muscles must be completely relaxed so that the surgeon can manipulate the fracture frag-ments to obtain reduction. This condition is obtained either with general anesthesia and muscle relaxants or with a successful regional interscalene block.

In the case of a two-part surgical neck fracture, or a three-part fracture in which there is significant displacement of the shaft from under the humeral head, a trial reduction is performed to confirm the feasibility of closed reduction and percutaneous fixation before sterile preparation and draping of the patient's arm. If the shaft cannot be reduced under the humeral head, the fracture pattern may be unstable or there is interposed soft tissue, and open reduction is indicated.

In many patients, the humeral shaft is either angulated with the apex anterior or completely displaced anteriorly as a result of the pull of the pectoralis major tendon. Reduction is performed by applying longitudinal traction with the arm in minimal abduction and some flexion (Figure 8). This position will relax tension on the pectoralis major, and posterior pressure on the humeral shaft may then reduce both displacement and angulation between the shaft and the humeral head fragments.

FIGURE 6

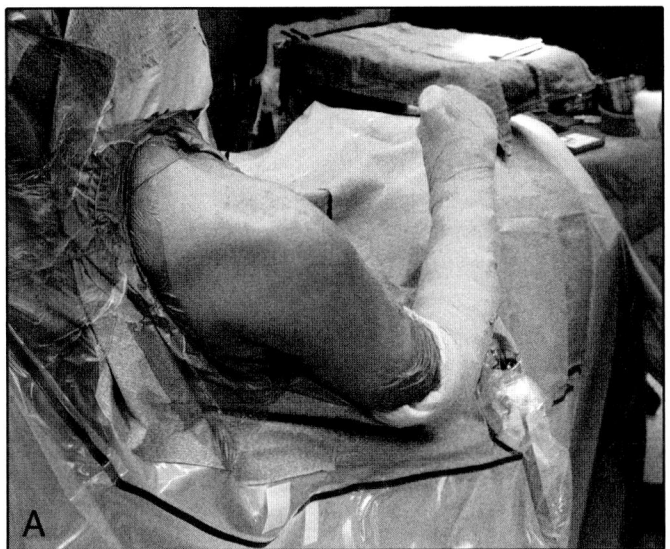

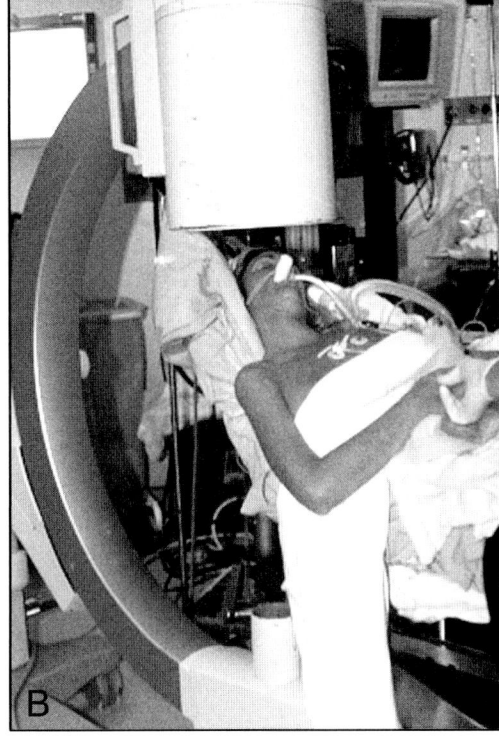

A, Positioning of a patient on a special beach chair (T-Max, Tenet Medical Engineering, Calgary, Canada) that allows full exposure of the shoulder for fluoroscopy. **B,** Positioning of a patient on a long beanbag contoured medial to the scapula so that the entire shoulder girdle is freely exposed for fluoroscopic biplanar imaging.

When closed reduction is confirmed, the shoulder and arm are sterilely prepared and an articulated arm holder is used to support and position the arm during the procedure (Figure 7). This arm holder permits reproducible, consistent positioning of the arm and allows the assistant to help with the fixation of the fracture.

Percutaneous Fixation With Pins

Two-Part Surgical Neck Fracture

In a two-part surgical neck fracture, the reduction maneuver is repeated as described, then the shaft is fixed to the articular segment as follows (Figure 9): A 2.5-mm terminally threaded pin is held over the shoulder, and a fluoroscopic AP image is obtained. The pin is positioned over the humeral head, coming from the lateral humeral shaft up into the head. The angle of the pin is marked with a skin marker on the shoulder. A small incision is then made over the lateral arm at the level determined by the fluoroscopic image, and a straight clamp is used to spread the soft-tissue down to the

humeral shaft. The tip of the clamp can confirm the anterior and posterior cortex of the humerus. The 2.5-mm terminally threaded pin is then positioned at this location through the small stab incision and confirmed with a fluoroscopic image. It is helpful to insert the pin into the lateral humeral cortex at a more horizontal angle so that the pin will not initially skate off the lateral cortex, which makes the angle more vertical. While the assistant maintains the reduction, the surgeon drills the pin up into the humeral head, confirming pin position with either spot radio-graphs or fluoroscopic control until the pin tip is just beneath the articular surface. Because the humeral shaft is in 20° of retrotorsion, the pin should be aligned in this orientation as it is inserted. The drill then is removed from the pin, and the shoulder is rotated while fluoroscopic imaging confirms that the pin is in the proper position. An axillary view should be obtained; however, simply rotating the shoulder into internal and external rotation will give a relatively quick and accurate assessment of pin placement.

A second pin is drilled parallel to the first pin so that

FIGURE 7

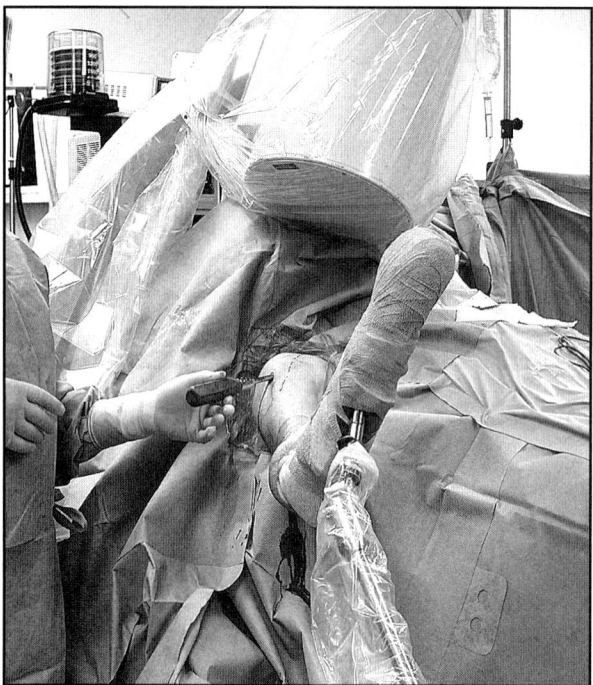

Positioning of a patient with the fluoroscope in position. The C-arm is draped with a sterile material and positioned at the head of the operating table. The arm is supported with a sterile, articulated arm holder (Spyder, Tenet Medical Engineering, Calgary, Canada).

FIGURE 8

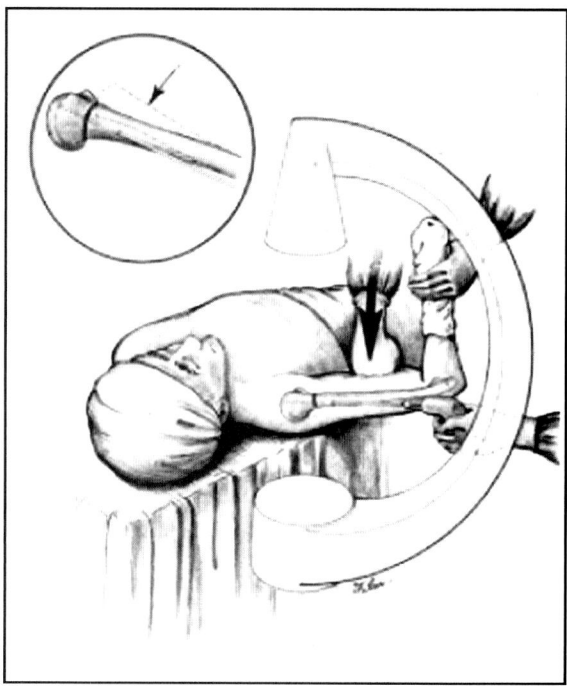

Closed reduction maneuver accomplished with distraction, flexion, and abduction. *(Reproduced with permission from Jaberg H, Warner JJ, Jakob RP: Percutaneous stabilization of unstable fractures of the humerus.* J Bone Joint Surg Am *1992;74:508-515.)*

the two pins are spread apart (ideally, 1.5 to 2.0 cm) in the humeral head. Finally, a third pin is placed through a small stab incision located anterior to the first incision so that this pin will enter the humeral head from an anterior direction. If necessary, a fourth pin can be added from an anterior direction for additional stability.

In some patients, an antegrade pin that enters from the greater tuberosity into the humeral shaft may be necessary. However, we have found this rarely to be the case in two-part surgical neck fractures.

Avoiding Pitfalls

The danger zones for pinning are the axillary nerve, which passes approximately 5 cm distal to the lateral edge of the acromion from posterior to anterior, and the radial nerve, which passes around the spiral groove of the humerus. The orientation of the lateral pins almost always is below the axillary nerve and above the radial nerve; however, we always spread the soft tissue down to

bone with a small clamp before placing the pin into the incision.

Anteriorly, the long head of the biceps tendon is a relative surgical danger, and medially, the anterior circumflex humeral vessels along the medial cortex also are considered a relative danger area.

It is imperative to obtain biplanar images during the procedure to assess pin placement in the humeral head, thereby avoiding penetration into the joint.

Three-Part Valgus-Impacted Fracture

In a three-part valgus-impacted fracture, the humeral articular fragment is tilted down into valgus, and the greater tuberosity remains at the correct height. The surgeon can use an indirect reduction maneuver, which takes advantage of soft-tissue tension in the rotator cuff and periosteum, to reduce the articular and greater tuberosity segments. Once the shaft has been positioned under the articular segment as described, a small inci-

FIGURE 9

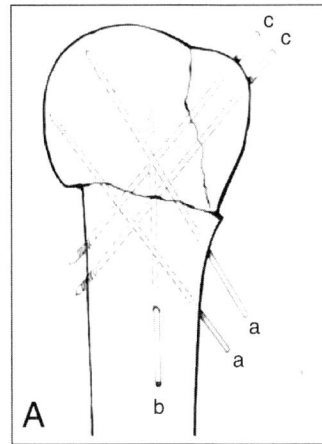
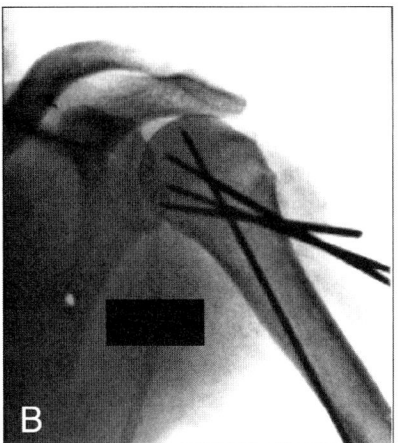
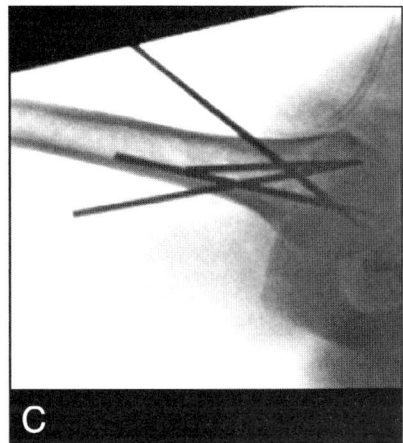

A, Percutaneous pin fixation technique. *(Reproduced with permission from Jaberg H, Warner JJ, Jakob RP: Percutaneous stabilization of unstable fractures of the humerus.* J Bone Joint Surg Am *1992;74:508-515.)* AP **(B)** and axillary **(C)** radiographs showing closed reduction and percutaneous pinning, demonstrating the retrograde technique with 2.5-mm terminally threaded pins. *(Courtesy of Christian Gerber, MD).*

sion is made laterally at a point that will allow an elevator to be placed into the fracture under the humeral head. The humeral head is then levered upward out of valgus and into proper varus alignment. This maneuver can be done under fluoroscopic control and should be very gentle so as not to risk fracturing the humeral articular segment. As the humeral head is tilted up out of valgus, the rotator cuff and periosteum will pull the greater tuberosity under the humeral articular segment, and in some patients, this will be an obvious reduction. While the surgeon holds this reduction in place, the assistant makes a small lateral incision above the first incision and places either 2.5-mm terminally threaded pins from the greater tuberosity or guidewires from the 4.0-mm cannulated screw set into the humeral head (Figure 10). The cannulated drill can be placed over the guide wires so that 4.0-mm screws of proper length can be used to fix the greater tuberosity to the articular segment, avoiding placement of pins through the rotator cuff and proximal deltoid. Several cannulated screws or pins should be used to fix the greater tuberosity to the humeral shaft in an antegrade orientation.

Four-Part Fracture
It occasionally may be possible to fix a four-part fracture in young patients with good quality bone using these techniques. The reduction and fixation of the humeral shaft and the greater tuberosity to the articu-

lar segment are performed as described. In patients in whom the greater tuberosity remains superiorly or posteriorly displaced, a 2.5-mm pin can be used as a joystick to manipulate the fragment into place so that it can be fixed to the humeral segment. Small hooks also can be used to accomplish the reduction (Figure 11).

The lesser tuberosity fragment also may require reduction, which is performed by internally rotating the arm and using a small hook placed through a small lateral incision to pull this fragment into position over the anterior humeral shaft. It is then fixed with 4.0-mm cannulated screws.

In all patients, final biplanar images should confirm reduction in both the AP and axillary planes. Some degree of malreduction of the shaft to the humeral head segment is acceptable as long as the configuration is stable; however, the tuberosities must be reduced into an anatomic position to avoid loss of motion resulting from malunion and mechanical blockage.

Aftercare
The pins are trimmed so that they are below the skin, which is closed with monofilament suture. The pins may become prominent as the swelling from the original injury subsides; therefore, the pins should be monitored to ensure that skin penetration is not imminent. If a pin penetrates the skin, it can be trimmed on an outpatient basis. The patient remains in the hospital overnight, and

FIGURE 10

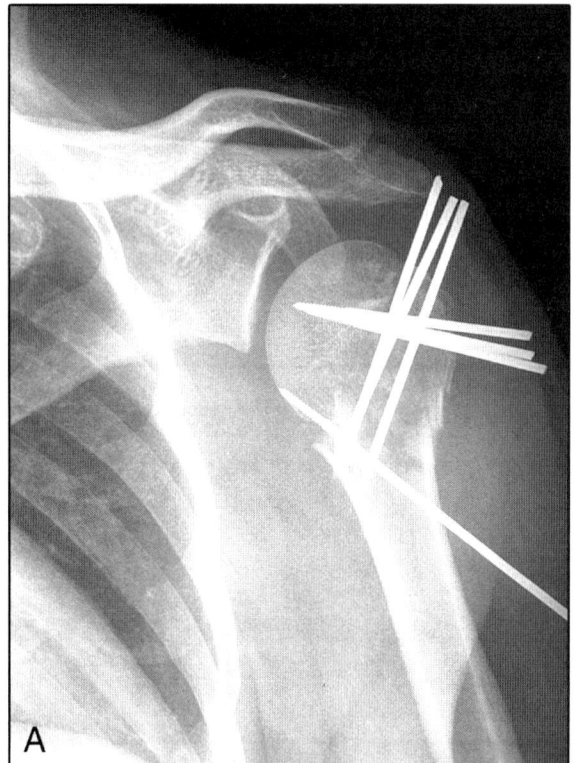

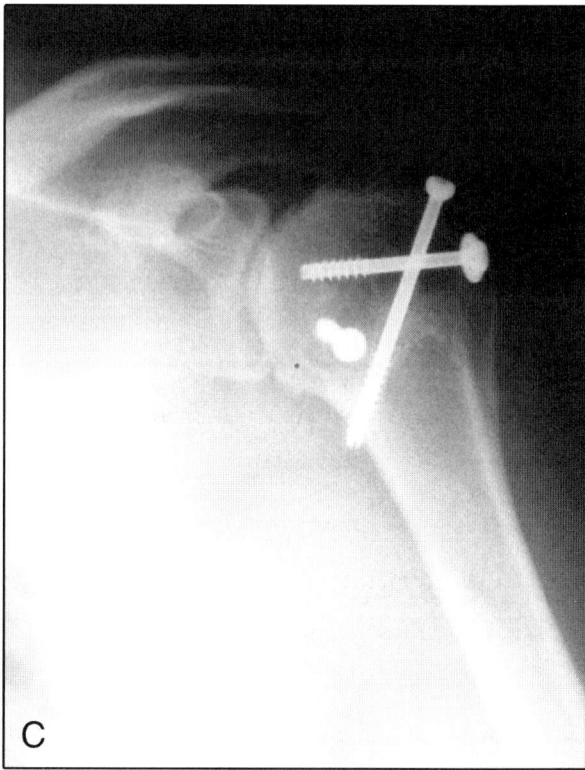

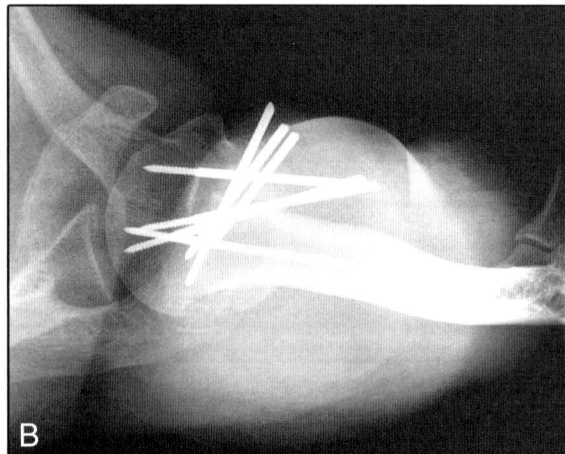

Postoperative AP **(A)** and axillary **(B)** radiographs of a three-part valgus-impacted fracture demonstrating anatomic reduction and fixation with 2.5-mm terminally threaded pins. **C,** Postoperative AP radiograph 2 years after closed reduction and percutaneous fixation of a four-part fracture with cannulated screws. Notice anatomic fracture union and no evidence of osteonecrosis. *(Courtesy of Evan Flatow, MD)*

prophylactic parenteral antibiotics are administered for the first 24 hours postoperatively.

The shoulder is placed into an immobilizer, and no motion is permitted for 4 weeks. However, if fixation has been achieved using cannulated screws so that no

pins are placed from an antegrade proximal position adjacent to the acromion, pendulum exercises are permitted in the first week after surgery.

A plan is made to return to the ambulatory operating room 4 to 6 weeks after the initial surgery to remove the

FIGURE 11

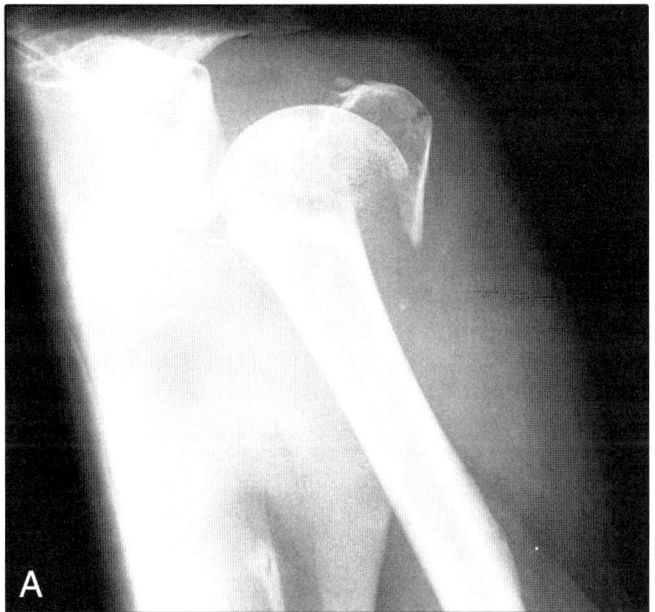

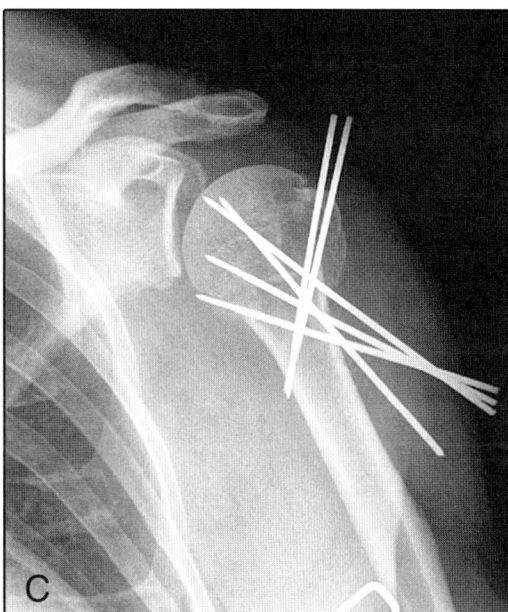

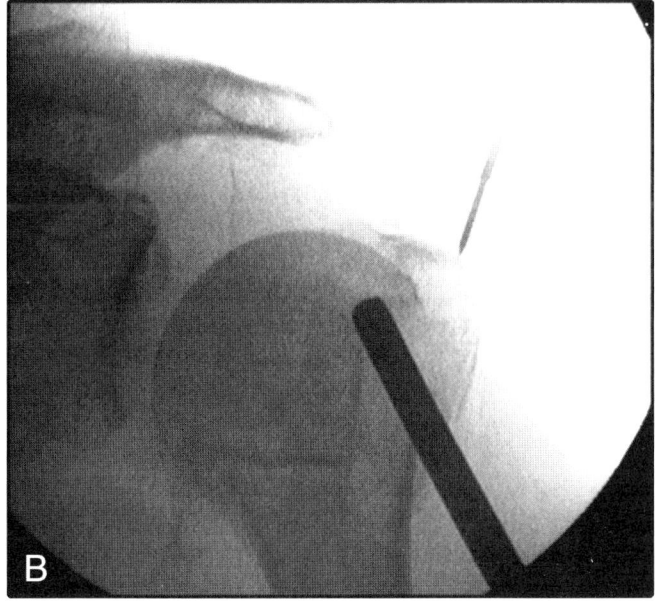

A, Valgus-impacted fracture. **B,** Mechanism of percutaneous reduction using a bone tamp to elevate the humeral head and a pin to joystick the greater tuberosity into place. **C,** Pinning after closed reduction.

provisional pin fixation. The patient is evaluated in the physician's office each week to check the pins, and biplanar images are obtained to ensure that pin migration has not occurred and that fracture reduction is maintained.

When the pins are removed, the patient begins active-assisted motion in a supervised physical therapy program. An aquatherapy program in which the patient is instructed to stretch the shoulder actively in a gravity-free buoyant environment of warm water also assists recovery of motion. Ideally, the patient should see a

FIGURE 12

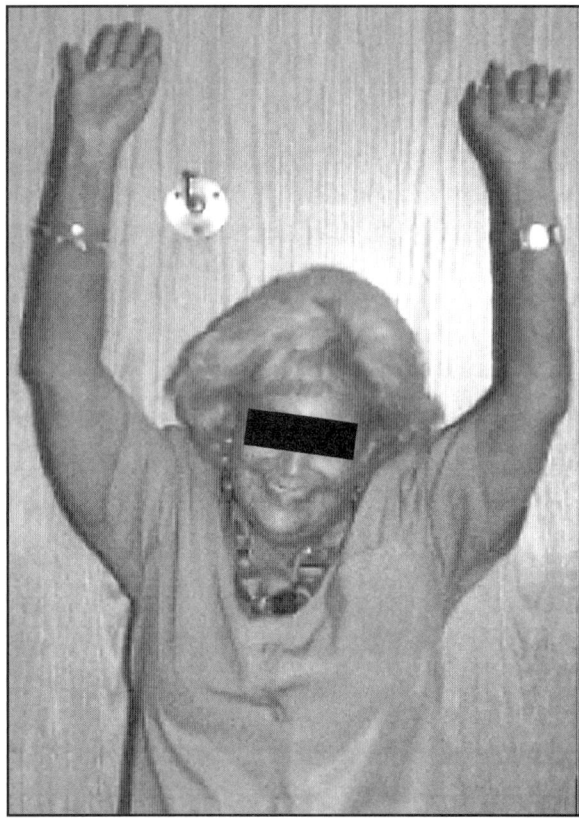

Final clinical result after closed reduction and percutaneous fixation of a three-part valgus-impacted fracture.

physical therapist three times each week for the first 4 to 6 weeks after surgery and attend aquatherapy at least twice a week after the pins are removed and the incision has healed. Using this approach, residual motion loss is rarely problematic.

Radiographs are obtained at 2 or 3 months after surgery, at which time complete radiographic union usually is apparent. Strengthening of the shoulder usually is begun at about 3 months after surgery.

RESULTS

The results of closed reduction and percutaneous pinning are favorable in most series.[3-6,8-11] The largest two series have been published by Jaberg and associates[3] and Resch and associates.[4,6]

Jaberg and associates[3] treated 54 unstable proximal humerus fractures with follow-up of 2 to 7 years (mean, 3 years). Of the 48 patients available for follow-up, 34 had a good or excellent result, 10 had a fair result, and 4 a poor result (loss of fixation). Osteonecrosis developed in two patients, and partial osteonecrosis developed in eight. This series was the first that inspired enthusiasm for this technique.

In 1997, Resch and associates[4] reported their experience treating the more complex patterns of three- and four-part fractures with closed reduction and percutaneous pinning. In this series, 27 patients were treated: 9 had three-part fractures, and 18 had four-part fractures, 13 of which were valgus impacted. Average follow-up was 2 years. The Constant score for three-part fractures was 91%, and no patients had osteonecrosis. For four-part fractures, the Constant score was 87%; however, 11% had osteonecrosis, and two patients required revision to a prosthesis for persistent pain.

In a follow-up study, Resch and associates[6] performed closed reduction and percutaneous fixation on 88 patients. The initial 27 patients (9 with type B1 and B2 fractures and 18 with type C1 and C2 fractures) were reported in follow-up. The type B1 and B2 fractures had a Constant score of 91%, indicating good to very good functional results; the type C1 and C2 fractures had a Constant score of 87% and an osteonecrosis rate of 11%. The authors concluded that the soft-tissue bridging of the various fragments was crucial for the reduction to benefit from the ligamentotaxis effect, and that this technique worked well for valgus-impacted or three-part fractures. The rate of osteonecrosis was low, and rehabilitation was easier because of limited adhesions within the surrounding tissues. Overall, the results from these series are quite encouraging.

Over the past 5 years, we have performed closed reduction and percutaneous fixation of 16 proximal humerus fractures. All patients have regained overhead motion and have achieved stable fixation (Figure 12). No osteonecrosis was observed; however, none of our patients had true four-part fractures.

PITFALLS AND FAILURES

Common pitfalls usually result from surgeon error and include inappropriate patient selection, inadequate reduction, convergence of pins, use of too few pins, or use of smooth pins with loss of reduction (Figure 13).

FIGURE 13

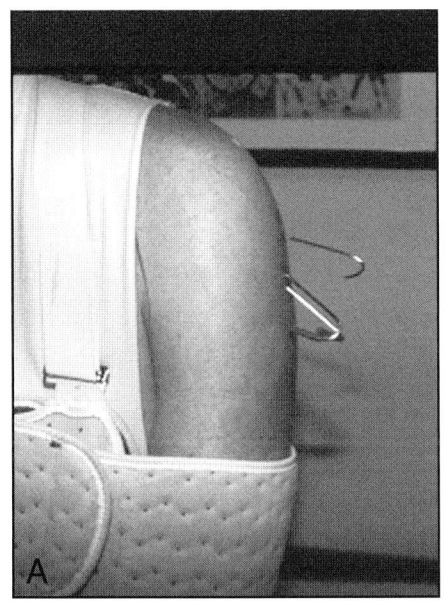
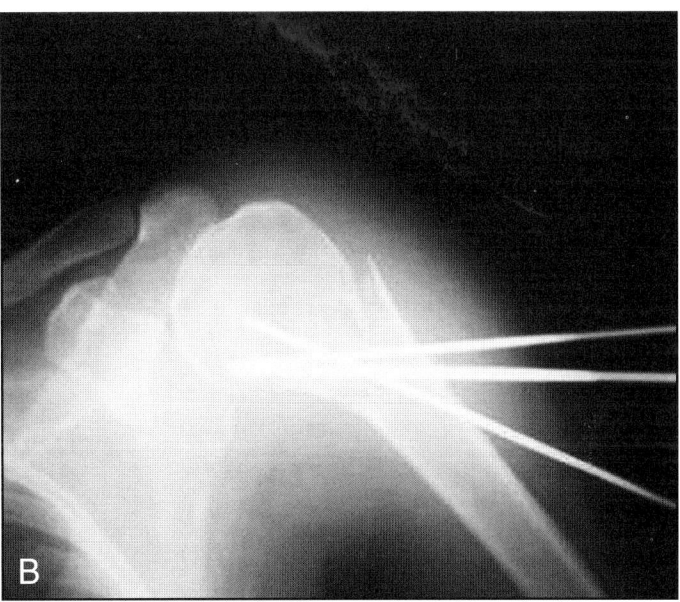

Technical errors associated with pin placement. **A,** Too few pins that were smooth and were left outside the skin. A pin tract infection developed in this patient. **B,** The pins were not widely displaced in the humeral head but instead were placed in a converging pattern into the articular segment. This led to a fracture nonunion.

Other causes include loss of reduction caused by failure to recognize comminution at the fracture site and pin tract infection caused by leaving pins outside the skin after the procedure.[13,14]

CONCLUSION

Closed reduction and percutaneous fixation is a useful technique in select patients with unstable proximal humerus fractures. Although the technique is demanding, the results are predictably good if meticulous attention is paid to the reduction and fixation steps. Furthermore, the biologic rationale of minimizing soft-tissue dissection to preserve articular vascularity is a very sound reason to select this approach in some three- and four-part fractures. The surgeon should develop skill and confidence with the technique with two-part fractures and then move to the more difficult three- and four-part fractures as his or her skills improve. The keys to success are proper setup, a careful reduction to restore the anatomy, a biomechanically sound pin configuration to maximize fixation, appropriate aftercare to achieve healing, and avoidance of complications.

REFERENCES

1. Gerber C, Warner JJP: Alternatives to hemiarthroplasty for complex proximal humeral fractures, in Warner JJP, Iannotti JP, Gerber C (eds): *Complex and Revision Problems in Shoulder Surgery.* Philadelphia, PA, Lippincott, Williams & Wilkins, 1997, pp 215-243.
2. Bohler J: Les fractures recentes de l'epaule. *Acta Orthop Belg* 1964;30:235.
3. Jaberg H, Warner JJ, Jakob RP: Percutaneous stabilization of unstable fractures of the humerus. *J Bone Joint Surg Am* 1992;74:508-515.
4. Resch H, Povacz P, Frohlich R, Wambacher M: Percutaneous fixation of three- and four-part fractures of the proximal humerus. *J Bone Joint Surg Br* 1997;79:295-300.
5. Herscovici D Jr, Saunders DT, Johnson MP, Sanders R, DiPasquale T: Percutaneous fixation of proximal humeral fractures. *Clin Orthop* 2000;375:97-104.
6. Resch H, Hubner C, Schwaiger R: Minimally invasive reduction and osteosynthesis of articular fractures of the humeral head. *Injury* 2001;32(suppl 1):SA25-SA32.
7. Gerber C, Schneeberger AG, Vinh TS: The arterial vascularization of the humeral head: An anatomical study. *J Bone Joint Surg Am* 1990;72:1486-1494.

8. Chen CY, Chao EK, Tu YK, Ueng SW, Shih CH: Closed management and percutaneous fixation of unstable proximal humerus fractures. *J Trauma* 1998;45:1039-1045.

9. Ebraheim N, Wong FY, Biyani A: Percutaneous pinning of the proximal humerus. *Am J Orthop* 1996;25:500-506.

10. Kocialkowski A, Wallace WA: Closed percutaneous K-wire stabilization for displaced fractures of the surgical neck of the humerus. *Injury* 1990;21:209-212.

11. Soete PJ, Clayson PE, Costenoble VH: Transitory percutaneous pinning in fractures of the proximal humerus. *J Shoulder Elbow Surg* 1999;8:569-573.

12. Williams GR Jr, Wong KL: Two-part and three-part fractures: Open reduction and internal fixation versus closed reduction and percutaneous pinning. *Orthop Clin North Am* 2000; 31:1-21.

13. Naidu SH, Bixler B, Capo JT, Moulton MJ, Radin A: Percutaneous pinning of proximal humerus fractures: A biomechanical study. *Orthopedics* 1997;20:1073-1076.

14. Rowles DJ, McGrory JE: Percutaneous pinning of the proximal part of the humerus: An anatomic study. *J Bone Joint Surg Am* 2001;83:1695-1699.

Open Reduction and Internal Fixation of Two- and Three-part Fractures

Matthew T. Boes, MD
Maryangela Moutoussis
Frances Cuomo, MD

Treatment of displaced two- and three-part proximal humerus fractures continues to be challenging. Options ranging from nonsurgical care to anatomic repair using various forms of internal fixation or prosthetic replacement are all well described.[1] Most proximal humerus fractures present as nondisplaced or minimally displaced, and several studies report acceptable functional outcomes when treated nonsurgically.[2-4] However, certain injuries tend to have a poorer outcome with nonsurgical treatment. These include fracture-dislocations, intra-articular fractures, and fractures in which significant displacement of the fracture fragments precludes healing in a functional position.[5,6] Interposed soft-tissue, deforming muscle forces, and disruption of the articular surface necessitate surgical intervention to adequately restore anatomic relationships and improve the potential for optimal function. Stable fixation that allows for early mobilization and adherence to a prolonged physician-directed rehabilitation program is required for any surgical treatment plan. Results following surgical management of two- and three-part fractures are maximized by accurate preoperative diagnosis, assessment of various patient factors, careful surgical technique, and attention to structured postoperative rehabilitation.

Classification

Several different classification systems have been proposed for proximal humerus fractures. In 1896, Kocher[7] described a system based on the anatomy of the fracture. Codman[8] was first to report that most fractures of the proximal humerus yielded four consistent anatomic fragments: the humeral head, humeral shaft, greater tuberosity, and lesser tuberosity. The four-part classification described by Neer[3,4] in 1970 remains the most commonly used and widely accepted description of these injuries. Fragments are defined by displacement greater than 1 cm or angulation greater than 45° from their anatomic position. Neer's classification is a refinement of Codman's system, which highlights the importance of both the biomechanical forces causing fragment displacement and the tenuous vascular supply of the articular fragment.[9]

CLINICAL EVALUATION

Assessment of a patient with a displaced fracture of the proximal humerus begins with a comprehensive examination for associated injuries. Patients will describe discomfort localized to the proximal limb that may supercede symptoms of injuries to other areas. It is essential to rule out associated injuries both to the involved extremity and to more distant areas. Significant shoulder injuries will produce a large amount of swelling and ecchymosis. Skin should be carefully examined to exclude open fracture. In addition, a careful neurovascular examination of the involved extremity should be performed to identify any deficits associated with the injury. Particular areas of concern include axillary nerve dysfunction and evidence of brachial plexopathy.[10] Examination of distal vascular perfusion and comparison of distal pulses helps identify associated vascular injury. Vascular injuries most commonly occur in the third part of the axillary artery where the vessel is tethered to the humerus by the anterior and posterior humeral circumflex branches. A significant medial shaft displacement through a surgical neck fracture is often apparent when vascular injury is present.[11,12] If a vascular injury is suspected, arteriography should be considered to document the level and extent of injury as well as to guide further treatment before undertaking definitive fracture fixation.

Proximal humerus fractures may occur in patients of all ages. Assessment of various patient factors and how they affect fracture management is essential to obtaining an optimal result. Factors such as patient age and physiologic level of function, medical comorbidities, and history of medication use may affect bone quality and, therefore, options for surgical fixation. An assessment of a patient's preinjury functional level helps tailor treatment goals for that patient.

The patient's arm may be placed in a sling at the time of clinical evaluation to provide gentle immobilization before undertaking definitive management. Gravity causes gentle traction on the fracture, which may reduce muscle spasm and provide relative stabilization of the fragments, leading to improved pain control. Patients should be advised to sleep in a semireclined position to decrease discomfort.

IMAGING

Accurate identification of the size, location, and displacement of the fragments is essential for fracture classification and formulation of a treatment plan. The initial radiographic study should be the trauma series consisting of the true AP, scapular lateral, and axillary views. This series has proved to be the most valuable in demonstrating the size and orientation of various fragments, as well as the magnitude and direction of their displacement.[13] The AP view identifies the major fracture lines; tuberosity and humeral head displacement are further defined on the lateral and axillary views. The axillary view predictably reveals the location of the articular surface in relation to the glenoid and most accurately identifies the lesser tuberosity fragment when it is displaced anteromedially by the subscapularis, and it often can be obscured by overlap of the humeral head and glenoid on the AP view. In addition, the axillary view aids in evaluating posterior displacement of the greater tuberostiy and adds significantly more information leading to an accurate diagnosis than the scapular lateral view.[14,15] A Velpeau axillary view may be substituted for the standard axillary view in patients who are unable to tolerate the position necessary for an axillary radiograph.[16] It often is necessary to supervise the radiographic studies to ensure appropriate views are obtained to minimize the need for repeat radiographs.

In most patients, the routine trauma series provides all the information required to assess the nature of the fracture. Additional radiographs may be needed in cases involving disruption of the humeral head in indentation and head-splitting fractures or comminution and displacement in associated glenoid fractures. CT is better than plain radiographs alone for evaluating the articular surface. However, it has been reported to be less beneficial for evaluating the relationship of the tuberosities to the humeral head and shaft.[17]

TREATMENT

The goal of surgical management is sufficient restoration of the anatomy to ensure soft-tissue and osseous healing that will result in maximal extremity function.

Factors important in choosing the nature of internal fixation include the level of the fracture, size of the fragments, and quality of the bone. Several reports have highlighted the benefits of various techniques for limited fixation. These techniques minimize soft-tissue disruption and fragment stripping, leading to improved potential healing.[18-21] Passage of heavy nonabsorbable sutures or wires through the rotator cuff tendon insertion provides stronger fixation than passage only through bone, which is often osteoporotic. The addition of intramedullary nails and rods (when the fracture involves the surgical neck) is an excellent method of achieving fixation in two- and three-part fractures while minimizing soft-tissue disruption[14,19] (D Contreras, MD, et al, unpublished data presented at the American Academy of Orthopaedic Surgeons annual meeting, 1990). Use of a humeral blade plate can provide rigid fixation for surgical neck fractures in young patients with good bone quality. This rigid fixation enables early rehabilitation with subsequent reduction in scarring and adhesions. Plates may be prefabricated or fashioned using semitubular plates. The fracture line must be at a level that allows insertion of the blade into the greater tuberosity, and the blade should be inserted to within 1 to 1.5 cm of the subchondral bone of the humeral head. This method involves greater soft-tissue disruption, but it also provides secure fixation in the strong subchondral bone of the humeral head linked to bicortical fixation in the shaft of the proximal humerus.[9]

INDICATIONS

Specific surgical indications for proximal humerus fractures remain poorly defined. A single surgical technique is not appropriate for all patients, and treatment must be tailored to each specific situation. Three groups of factors must be considered when contemplating surgical treatment: surgeon factors, characteristics of the fracture, and condition of the patient. The surgeon must be able to make an accurate radiographic diagnosis and have a thorough knowledge of the anatomy of the shoulder girdle. Surgeon comfort level with various procedures may exclude certain techniques from consideration. Characteristics of the fracture also determine the type of management because certain injuries may not be amenable to a particular surgical approach or fixation technique. Last, the patient's general medical condition, physiologic age, and ability to comply with a demanding and prolonged rehabilitation program are important considerations.

Greater tuberosity fractures in which there is significant displacement of the fragment require surgical repair to prevent rotator cuff deficiency and/or subacromial impingement of the cuff tendons. Previously, displacement greater than 1 cm was considered significant, but more recently authors have reported that more than 0.5 cm of superior displacement may lead to pain or disability after fracture healing. Indications for surgical repair of lesser tuberosity fractures include fractures that involve a significant amount of the humeral head articular surface attached to the fragment or fractures that limit internal rotation of the shoulder. Two-part anatomic neck fractures, particularly in young patients, may be treated with open reduction and internal fixation (ORIF) if the size of the head fragment does not preclude secure fixation. Although preservation of the anatomic head should be attempted in younger patients, the tenuous blood supply to the humeral head places this fragment at risk for osteonecrosis following an anatomic neck fracture. In older patients, prosthetic replacement is often the best treatment for two-part anatomic neck fractures. Two-part surgical neck fractures that cannot be acceptably reduced because of deforming muscle forces or soft-tissue interposition are best managed surgically. In addition, fracture-dislocations involving the surgical neck and two-part tuberosity fracture-dislocations in which the tuberosities fail to adequately reduce following reduction of the dislocation also warrant open management. ORIF remains the treatment of choice for most three-part fractures unless advanced age or medical conditions have affected bone quality, making secure fixation difficult.

TECHNIQUE

Positioning

The techniques for stabilization of proximal humerus fractures are facilitated with use of the beach-chair or semireclining position in which the head and back are elevated 30°, and the knees are flexed. Bony prominences are carefully padded to prevent pressure injury. Hyperextension of the neck is avoided by carefully positioning the head to prevent injury to the cervical spine. Attention is directed at ensuring mobility of the

FIGURE 1

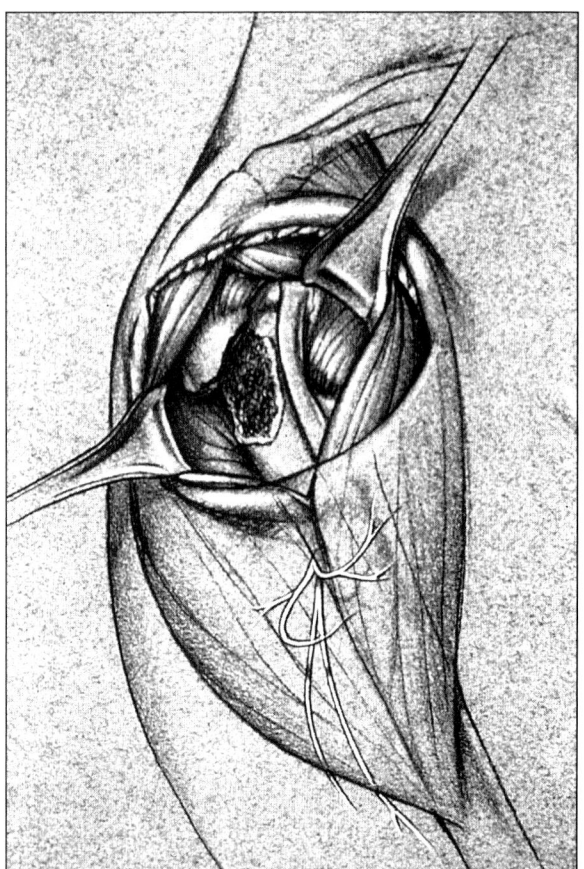

Skin incision for the deltoid-splitting approach extends 7 to 8 cm along Langer's lines just off the lateral margin of the acromion. A stay-suture is placed 4 to 5 cm from the acromion to avoid propagation of the split and injury to the axillary nerve. *(Reproduced with permission from Bigliani LU, Flatow EL, Pollock RG: Fractures of the proximal humerus, in Rockwood CA, Matsen FA (eds): The Shoulder, ed 2. Philadelphia, PA, Saunders, 1998, pp 337-389.)*

FIGURE 2

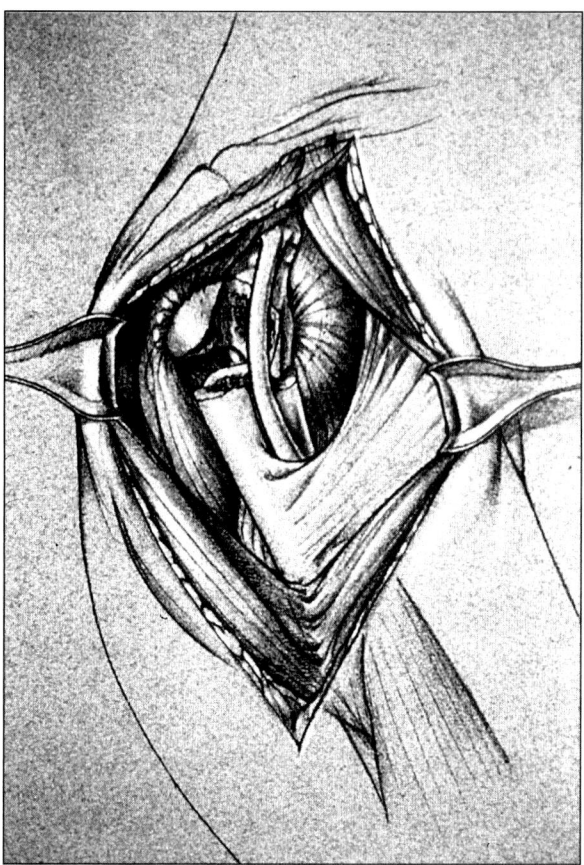

Deltopectoral approach. The skin incision begins at the level of the clavicle, crosses the lateral margin of the coracoid, and extends to the level of the deltoid insertion. Following deep dissection through the deltopectoral interval, the pectoralis major tendon may be released to facilitate exposure and fracture reduction. *(Reproduced with permission from Bigliani LU, Flatow EL, Pollock RG: Fractures of the proximal humerus, in Rockwood CA, Matsen FA (eds): The Shoulder, ed 2. Philadelphia, PA, Saunders, 1998, pp 337-389.)*

arm during the procedure to allow for reduction maneuvers and to enable insertion of fixation devices. The entire upper extremity is prepared and draped, with care taken to avoid excessive abduction of the arm, which risks injury to neurovascular structures from osseous spikes.

Surgical Exposure

Most two- and three-part proximal humeral fractures may be exposed using either a deltoid-splitting or a deltopectoral approach. The size and location of the frac-

ture fragments dictate which approach is used. Both approaches provide adequate exposure in appropriate patients while preserving the origin and insertion of the deltoid, which is critical to successful rehabilitation. Injury to the axillary nerve can be avoided with awareness of the nerve's course as it exits the quadrangular space and traverses the substance of the deltoid.

Deltoid-Splitting Approach
The deltoid-splitting, or superior, approach is most useful in the treatment of two-part greater tuberosity frac-

tures. The greater tuberosity fragment and rotator cuff may be mobilized and repaired through this approach without disrupting the deltoid origin. This approach also may be used to expose the insertion site for intramedullary nails in two-part surgical neck fractures. An incision is made immediately lateral to the anterolateral corner of the acromion in the direction of Langer's skin-tension lines (Figure 1). Superior and inferior skin flaps are elevated to allow mobility of the incision to provide greater exposure. Risk of injury to the axillary nerve in the distal portion of the deltoid split is decreased by placing a suture 4 to 5 cm from the leading edge of the acromion to prevent tension on the nerve. Subdeltoid adhesions are gently cleared using a Darrach retractor, and the deltoid is retracted to expose the greater tuberosity fracture bed. Bursal tissue and fracture hematoma are removed to clear the fracture bed and allow for anatomic reduction of the fragment. If the tuberosity fragment is retracted posteriorly, it can be retrieved by extending and internally rotating the arm to expose the fragment.

Deltopectoral Approach

The deltopectoral approach is a utilitarian approach that spares the deltoid origin and can be used to treat all two- and three-part surgical neck fractures. Landmarks for the incision, including the clavicle, coracoid, and deltoid tuberosity, are marked with the arm in neutral rotation. The incision begins at the level of the clavicle, extends over the lateral portion of the coracoid, and ends at the level of the deltoid insertion roughly adjacent to the proximal extent of the axilla (Figure 2). The deltopectoral interval is identified by the cephalic vein, which is mobilized while attempting to keep it intact. Because most of its feeder vessels enter from the deltoid side, the cephalic vein generally is more easily mobilized laterally, although it may be mobilized medially if that facilitates fracture exposure. The leading edge of the coracoacromial ligament may be resected to obtain superior visualization and mobilization of fragments. The pectoralis major tendon may be released to decrease its deforming force on the humeral shaft, which can complicate reduction of the fragments. If not already disrupted by the fracture fragments, the clavipectoral fascia is sharply entered adjacent to the conjoined tendon to allow retractors to gently distract the strap muscles medially and the deltoid laterally. Care should be taken to avoid excessive force on

these retractors because it can lead to traction injury to the nerves. Hemorrhagic bursae, clots, and fibrinous debris are excised fully, exposing the rotator cuff and proximal humerus.

Two-part Greater Tuberosity Fractures

Following a deltoid-splitting approach and débridement of the fracture bed, the tuberosity fragment is identified and mobilized using heavy nonabsorbable sutures inserted at the bone-tendon interface (Figure 3). Sutures incorporating the rotator cuff tendon insertions often are stronger than those placed in bone alone. The sutures should be placed at the levels of the superior, middle, and inferior facets of the greater tuberosity fragment to counteract the displacing forces of all components of the rotator cuff musculature. Fracture fragments may displace superiorly and/or posteriorly depending on the location of the fracture and the area of involvement of the tuberosity in relation to the cuff tendon insertions. It may be necessary to remove a small amount of cancellous bone from the undersurface of the fragment to facilitate reduction. Drill holes are made around the fracture bed for passage of fixation sutures (Figure 4).

A rotator cuff tear frequently can be associated with the fracture and located in the rotator interval or more posteriorly between the supraspinatus and infraspinatus. Repair of the rotator cuff tear is essential because the repaired rotator cuff holds the fracture fragment reduced. Repairing the tear after reducing the fragment but before fragment fixation will help remove tension from the tuberosity fixation. Next, the tuberosity is securely fixed to the shaft with heavy, nonabsorbable sutures through the previously placed drill holes and tied in a figure-of-eight fashion (Figure 5). Finally, the deltoid is closed using nonabsorbable sutures.

Two-part Lesser Tuberosity Fractures

Isolated, displaced lesser tuberosity fractures are rare.[22] ORIF is indicated when a significant amount of humeral head articular surface is attached to the fragment or when a block to internal rotation is present. These fractures are repaired similarly to greater tuberosity fractures. The pull of the subscapularis attached to the lesser tuberosity fragment often leads to anteromedial dis-

FIGURE 3

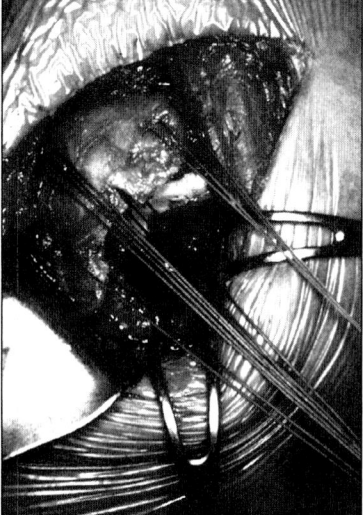

Suture placement in the bone-tendon junction for mobilization and reduction of the greater tuberosity fragment. Placement at the superior, middle, and inferior facets will correct both superior and posterior displacement. *(Reproduced with permission from Cuomo F, Zuckerman JD: Open reduction and internal fixation of two- and three-part proximal humeral fractures. Tech Orthop 1994;9:141-153.)*

FIGURE 4

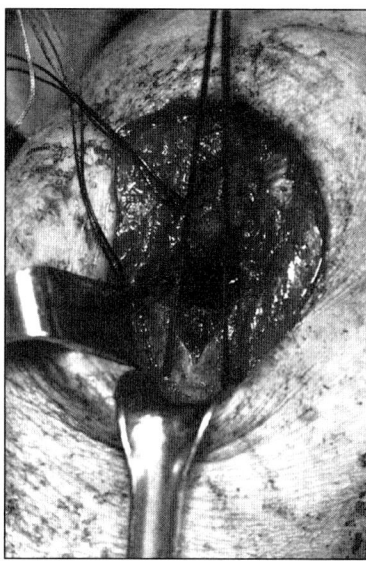

The fracture bed is débrided, and sutures are placed through drill holes around the periphery to ensure accurate reduction and secure fixation. *(Reproduced with permission from Cuomo F, Zuckerman JD: Open reduction and internal fixation of two- and three-part proximal humeral fractures. Tech Orthop 1994;9:141-153.)*

FIGURE 5

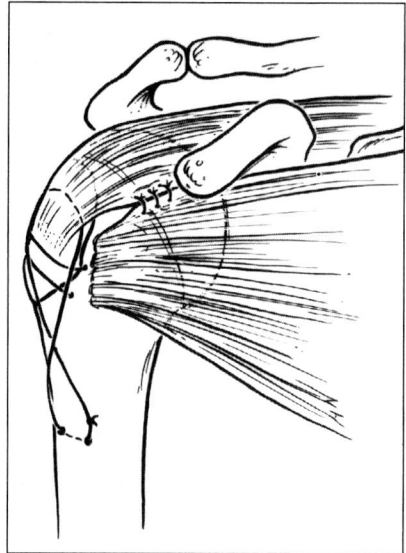

Diagram showing the greater tuberosity fragment reduced and secured with figure-of-eight sutures incorporating the bone-tendon interface of the rotator cuff tendons after closure of the rotator interval. *(Reproduced with permission from Cuomo F, Zuckerman JD: Open reduction and internal fixation of two- and three-part proximal humeral fractures. Tech Orthop 1994;9:141-153.)*

placement of the fragment. Exposure may, therefore, be best achieved by using a deltopectoral or anterior axillary approach.

The anterior axillary approach differs slightly from the standard deltopectoral approach in that the skin incision is vertical and made in the anterior axillary crease for better cosmesis. The skin and subcutaneous tissue must be undermined both superiorly and medially to gain mobility for exposure. The subsequent steps of this approach are similar to the deltopectoral approach.

External rotation and forward elevation of the arm improve visualization and isolation of the subscapularis and lesser tuberosity fragment. The lesser tuberosity fragment is then mobilized with heavy nonabsorbable sutures and reduced into the débrided fracture bed. Sutures placed through drill holes around the periphery of the bed are used to secure the fragment as previously described for the greater tuberosity. Excision of the bony fragment from the subscapularis and anterior capsule and reattachment of the subscapularis also have been described.[22]

Two-part Surgical Neck Fractures

Displaced surgical neck fractures are most easily exposed through a deltopectoral approach. The fracture site is cleared of hematoma and debris, and the head and shaft fragments are gently mobilized. The humeral head can be controlled by using traction sutures placed at the bone-tendon junction or by using bone reduction forceps to approximate the head to the shaft. Forward elevation of the arm while gently pulling on the sutures controlling the head will assist in reduction. The head fragment is then impacted on the shaft and the arm is brought toward a neutral position while maintaining tension on the sutures to hold the reduction (Figure 6).

The repair is made using heavy nonabsorbable

FIGURE 6

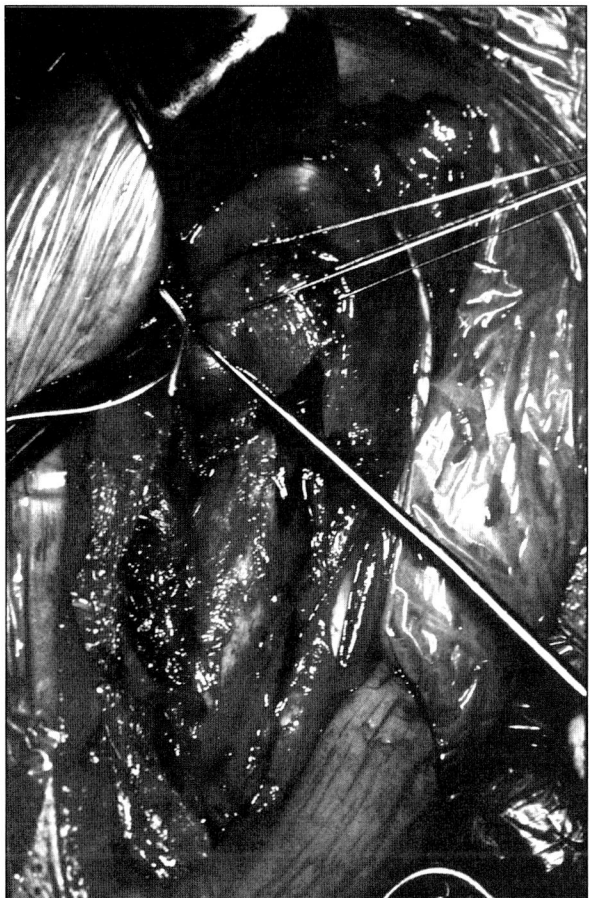

Sutures used to facilitate reduction of the head fragment to the shaft in a two-part surgical neck fracture.

sutures or wires secured through drill holes in the shaft in a figure-of-eight fashion. This construct may be supplemented with intramedullary or Ender-type nails in a tension-band configuration. Wires can provide greater stability but also can be associated with risks of breakage and irritation of adjacent soft tissues. Therefore, sutures are used to avoid these complications. The shallow bend of Ender nails (3.5 mm) offers three-point fixation of the fracture and, therefore, enhanced stability of the construct. In this sense, the nails provide greater stability than straight rods such as Rush rods, but both types of intramedullary devices help to prevent medial displacement of the shaft fragment. The combination of tension-band sutures or wires and

intramedullary fixation adds greater translational and rotational stability compared with either tension banding or intramedullary nailing alone (B Blair, MD, et al, unpublished data presented at the Orthopaedic Trauma Association annual meeting, 1993). This added fixation is particularly important when there is comminution of the fracture site and, therefore, less inherent stability from interdigitation of the fracture fragments.[19]

Small stab incisions are made in the direction of the rotator cuff fibers over the greater or lesser tuberosity just lateral to the articular surface nail insertion. In addition to the added stability, another benefit of Ender nails is the presence of the proximal eyelet in the nail that can accept figure-of-eight sutures or wires. Placement of a suture or wire through the eyelet prevents subsequent proximal migration of the nail leading to subacromial impingement[19] (D Contreras, MD, et al, unpublished data presented at the American Academy of Orthopaedic Surgeons annual meeting, 1990). Recent Ender nail designs are modified with a tiny suture hole located proximally to the standard oblong slot used for nail insertion. This proximal suture eyelet allows for deeper insertion of the nail into the humeral head, placing the tip well below the cuff tendons and reducing soft-tissue irritation[19] (Figure 7).

Sites for nail insertion depend on the location of fractures within the tuberosity. The greater tuberosity is generally large enough to accept two nails as opposed to only one in the smaller lesser tuberosity. If no fractures are present in the greater tuberosity to prevent secure nail placement, then two nails should be placed in the greater tuberosity just outside of the articular surface. After incisions are made through the supraspinatus tendon, a nail insertion hole is made in the tuberosity using an awl. It is helpful to place the posterior nail first because once it is partially inserted it can be used to lever the proximal fragment and aid in maintaining the reduction by preventing the humeral head from falling posteriorly (Figure 8).

The second nail is inserted approximately 1.0 to 1.5 cm anterior to the first. Use of nails of two different lengths may help prevent creation of a stress riser in the humeral shaft near the distal tip of the nails.[19] Before full seating of the nails, drill holes are made in the humeral shaft to accept tension-band sutures or wires, which are placed through the proximal eyelets of the nails and passed deep to the rotator cuff tendon between

FIGURE 7

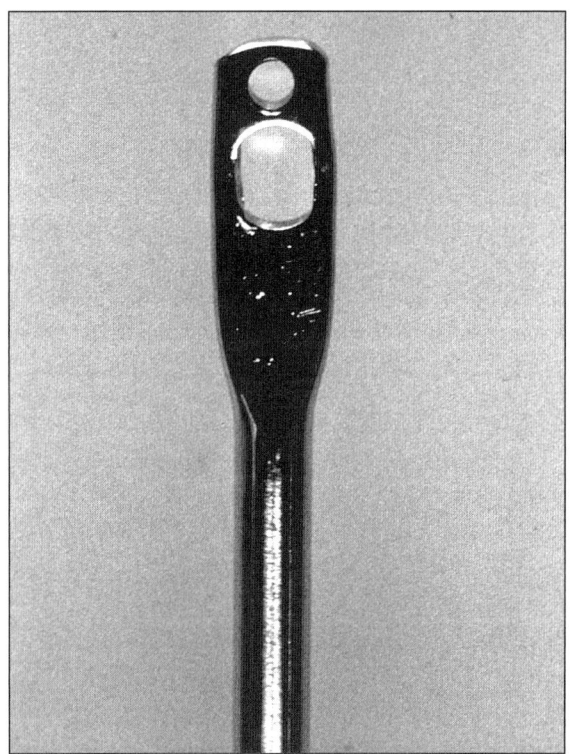

Modified Ender nail showing suture eyelet proximal to the oblong nail-insertion eyelet. *(Reproduced with permission from Cuomo F, Flatow EL, Maday MG, Miller SR, McIlveen SJ, Bigliani LU: Open reduction and internal fixation of two- and three-part displaced surgical neck fractures of the proximal humerus. J Shoulder Elbow Surg 1992;1:287-293.)*

FIGURE 8

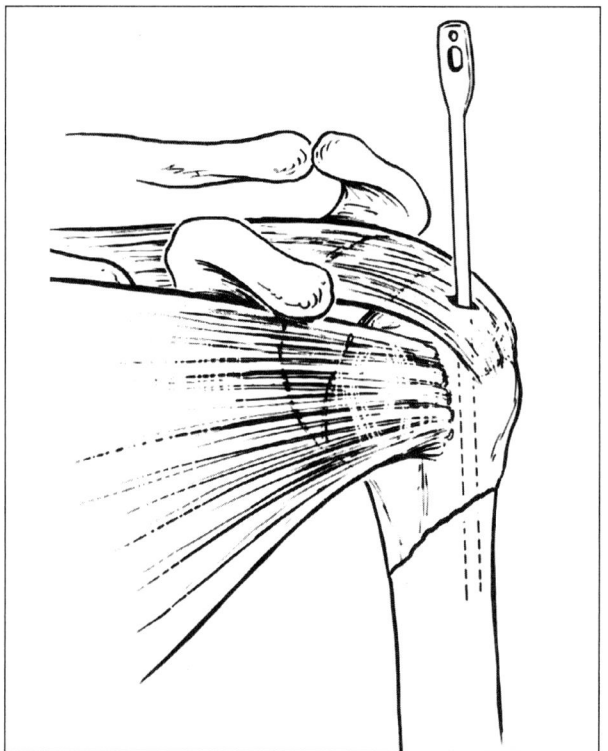

The posterior nail is introduced first in a two-part surgical neck fracture to assist in stabilizing the head fragment to the shaft. *(Reproduced with permission from Cuomo F, Zuckerman JD: Open reduction and internal fixation of two- and three-part proximal humeral fractures. Tech Orthop 1994;9:141-153.)*

the nails. The sutures or wires are then crossed in a figure-of-eight fashion and passed through the predrilled holes in the shaft (Figure 9, *A*). Nails are impacted well below the cuff, and fracture reduction is evaluated before tightening the tension band.

Finally, the stability of the fixation is assessed intraoperatively to establish safe parameters for postoperative rehabilitation and prevent subsequent stress on the repair. The cuff incisions are repaired, and the deltopectoral interval is closed in standard fashion. A closed suction drain is used depending on the drainage encountered (Figure 9, *B*).

Three-part Fractures

The disruption of normal anatomy associated with three-part fractures creates a significant treatment challenge. Knowledge of consistent anatomic landmarks and careful surgical technique can greatly simplify the procedure.

The deltopectoral approach provides a wide exposure through which all aspects of the injury may be addressed. The long head of the biceps tendon provides a consistent anatomic landmark for discerning the greater and lesser tuberosity fragments located laterally and medially to it, respectively. The biceps tendon is located deep to the pectoralis major insertion and should be protected if the pectoralis is released. Tracing the biceps proximally will lead to identification of the rotator interval, which is incised medially to the level of the glenoid to facilitate exposure and mobilization of the fracture fragments. The displaced tuberosity fragment is mobilized, as previously described, using heavy

FIGURE 9

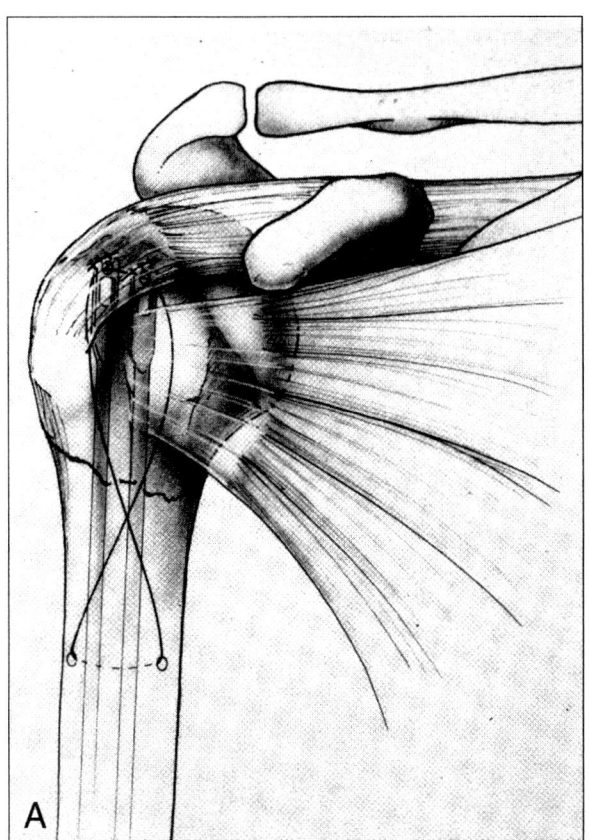
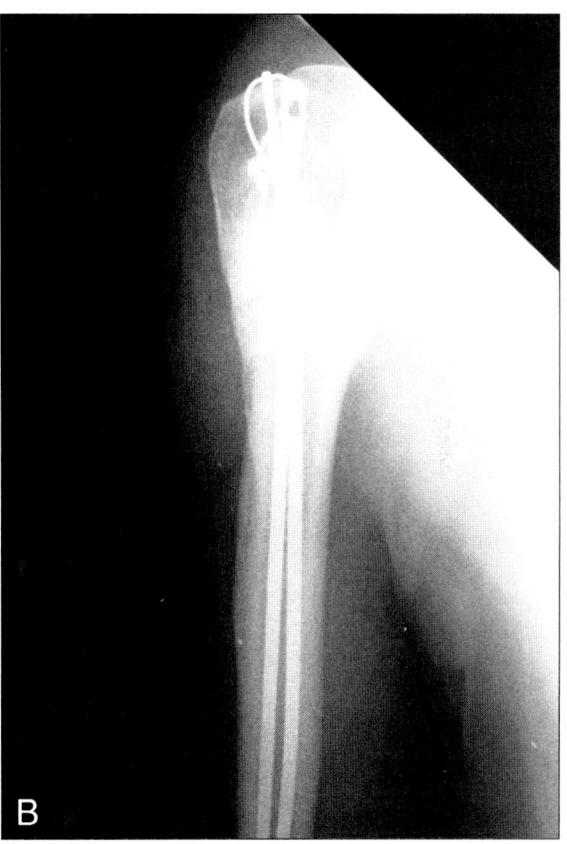

A, Two-part surgical neck fracture with Ender nail and tension-band suture fixation in place. The suture is passed through the suture eyelets in the nail and under the rotator cuff tendon, then the nails are fully seated to prevent tendon irritation. *(Reproduced with permission from Cuomo F, Flatow EL, Maday MG, Miller SR, McIlveen SJ, Bigliani LU: Open reduction and internal fixation of two- and three-part displaced surgical neck fractures of the proximal humerus.* J Shoulder Elbow Surg *1992;1:287-293.)* **B,** AP radiograph taken 6 months after repair of two-part surgical neck fracture using nail and tension-band technique.

nonabsorbable sutures. The humeral head fragment and its attached tuberosity may be mobilized similarly. A dislocated humeral head is controlled and reduced using traction sutures and a blunt Darrach retractor, or bone reduction forceps may be used to grasp the humeral head and gently bring it back into position. Care should be taken when reducing a humeral head fragment that is dislocated inferiorly and medially to the glenoid to prevent injury to neurovascular structures located inferomedially to the coracoid.

Following adequate control of all fragments, the tuberosity fragment is reduced first and secured to the head fragment using drill holes and heavy sutures (Fig-ure 10, *A*). This proximal construct is then reduced onto the shaft as previously described. Ender nails are inserted in the uninvolved tuberosity (two for the greater tuberosity, one for the lesser tuberosity) to stabilize the surgical neck fracture (Figure 10, *B* and *C*). Drill holes are placed in the shaft, both medially and laterally to the biceps tendon, for figure-of-eight fixation of both the tuberosity fragment and the humeral head. The involved tuberosity is thus secured to both the head fragment and the shaft fragment. The surgical neck fracture is repaired using tension banding and intramedullary nailing to the shaft, as previously described (Figure 10, *D*).

FIGURE 10

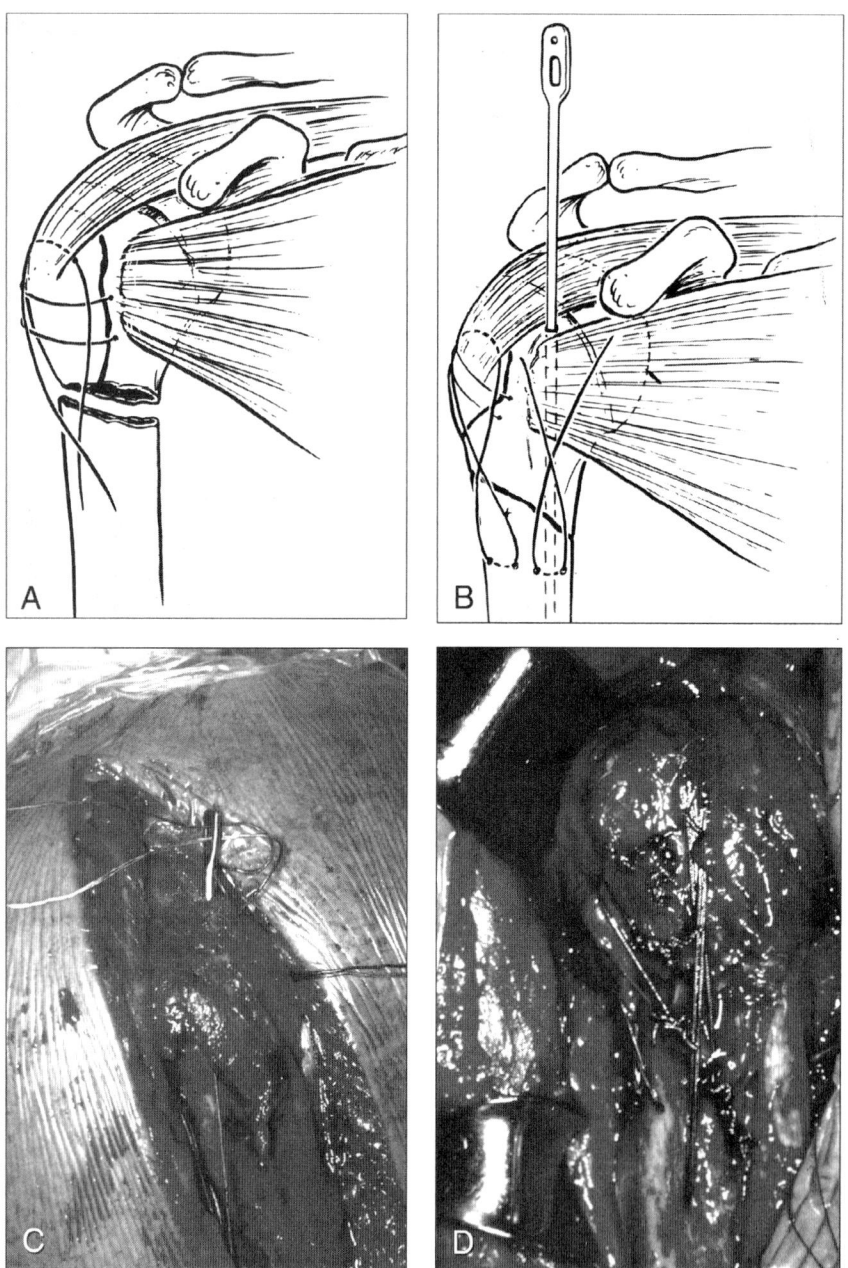

A, Diagram showing three-part greater tuberosity and surgical neck fracture. The tuberosity is fixed to the head fragment using multiple non-absorbable sutures converting a two-part to a three-part fracture. **B,** The secured tuberosity-head fragment unit is reduced and fixed to the shaft with a nail inserted through the intact lesser tuberosity. **C,** Intraoperative photograph showing Ender nail insertion with sutures placed through nail holes. **D,** Final fixation with proximal fragments secured to the shaft with multiple figure-of-eight tension-band sutures placed through drill holes in the proximal shaft. Exact fixation for each fracture type may vary with specific fracture geometry. *(Reproduced with permission from Cuomo F, Zuckerman JD: Open reduction and internal fixation of two- and three-part proximal humeral fractures. Tech Orthop 1994;9:141-153.)*

The stability of the fixation is evaluated intraoperatively, and stress-free limits on the repair are noted to assist in guiding postoperative rehabilitation. The rotator interval, cuff incisions, and deltopectoral interval are repaired as previously described.

REHABILITATION

Physician-supervised postoperative rehabilitation is vital for successful results following surgical treatment of displaced proximal humerus fractures. Patients should be advised preoperatively that maximal postoperative function may not be restored until up to 1 year after surgery. The goal of surgical repair is to allow early passive motion and active-assisted exercises. Early motion is a key factor in preventing formation of adhesions, which can limit motion postoperatively and can be challenging to overcome once they have developed.

Passive range-of-motion exercises usually are started immediately after surgery, specifically with pendulum exercises and passive forward elevation in the scapular plane. Depending on the security of the fixation as evaluated at the time of surgery, gentle external rotation at the side, assisted with a stick between both hands, is also begun in the early postoperative period. Once healing is noted at 6 to 8 weeks, active range-of-motion exercises followed by progressive strengthening exercises are begun.

CONCLUSION

ORIF of displaced two- and three-part proximal humerus fractures can be technically demanding. Difficulties may be minimized with a thorough understanding of the anatomy, accurate interpretation of appropriate radiographs, careful soft-tissue handling at the time of surgery, and secure and accurate reduction and fixation. Minimally disruptive fixation including the use of heavy, nonabsorbable sutures or wires and incorporating the strong rotator cuff tendons, tuberosities, and shaft is a sound method of achieving fixation and osseous union. Ender nails used in conjunction with figure-of-eight sutures or wires in a tension-band construct can provide additional stability in surgical neck fractures, especially if comminution exists. Fixation of this type helps to minimize the complications of soft-tissue stripping and loss of fixation in osteoporotic bone while permitting the institution of an early passive range-of-motion rehabilitation program essential for achieving optimal results. Failure to institute and maintain a supervised rehabilitation program in the immediate postoperative period will likely undermine surgical results despite restoration of anatomy and secure fixation.

REFERENCES

1. Bigliani LU, Flatow EL, Pollock RG: Fractures of the proximal humerus, in Rockwood CA, Matsen FA, Wirth MA, Harryman D (eds): *The Shoulder*, ed 2. New York, NY, WB Saunders, 1998, pp 337-390.

2. Koval KJ, Gallagher MA, Marsicano JG, et al: Functional outcome after minimally displaced fractures of the proximal part of the humerus. *J Bone Joint Surg Am* 1997;79:203-207.

3. Neer CS II: Displaced proximal humeral fractures: Part II. Treatment of three and four part displacement. *J Bone Joint Surg Am* 1970;52:1090-1103.

4. Neer CS II: Displaced proximal humeral fractures: Part I. Classification and evaluation. *J Bone Joint Surg Am* 1970;52:1077-1089.

5. Kristiansen B, Christensen SW: Plate fixation of proximal humeral fractures. *Acta Orthop Scand* 1987;57:320-323.

6. Mouradian WH: Displaced proximal humeral fractures: Seven years' experience with a modified Zickel supracondylar device. *Clin Orthop* 1986;212:209-218.

7. Kocher T: Beitrage zur kenntnis Einiger Praktisch Wichtiger Fracturenformen. Basel, Switzerland, Carl Sallman Verlag, 1896.

8. Codman EA: *Rupture of the Supraspinatus Tendon and Other Lesions In or About the Subacromial Bursa*. Boston, MA, Thomas Todd, 1934.

9. Williams GR, Wong KL: Two-part and three-part fractures: Open reduction and internal fixation versus closed reduction and percutaneous pinning. *Orthop Clin North Am* 2000;31:1-21.

10. Blom S, Dahlback LO: Nerve injuries in dislocations of the shoulder joint and fractures of the neck of the humerus: A clinical and electromyographical study. *Acta Chir Scand* 1970;136:461-466.

11. Bigliani LU: Fractures of the proximal humerus, in Rockwood CA, Matsen FA (eds): *The Shoulder*. New York, NY, WB Saunders, 1990, p 278-319.

12. Stableforth PG: Four-part fractures of the neck of the humerus. *J Bone Joint Surg Br* 1984;66:104-108.

13. Neer CS II, Rockwood CA: Fractures and dislocations of the shoulder, in Rockwood CA, Green DP (eds): *Fractures in Adults.* Philadelphia, PA, Lippincott, 1984, pp 675-721.

14. Flatow EL, Cuomo F, Maday MG, Miller SR, McIlveen SJ, Bigliani LU: Open reduction and internal fixation of two-part displaced fractures of the greater tuberosity of the proximal part of the humerus. *J Bone Joint Surg Am* 1991;73:1213-1218.

15. Sidor ML, Zuckerman JD, Lyon T, Koval K, Schoenberg N: Classification of proximal humerus fractures: The contribution of the scapular lateral and axillary radiographs. *J Shoulder Elbow Surg* 1994;3:24-27.

16. Bloom MH, Obata WG: Diagnosis of posterior dislocation of the shoulder with use of Velpeau axillary and angle-up roentgenographic views. *J Bone Joint Surg Am* 1967;49:943-949.

17. Sidor ML, Zuckerman JD, Lyon T, et al: The Neer classification system for proximal humeral fractures: An assessment of interobserver reliability and intraobserver reproducibility. *J Bone Joint Surg Am* 1993;75:1745-1750.

18. Cofield RH: Comminuted fractures of the proximal humerus. *Clin Orthop* 1988;230:49-57.

19. Cuomo F, Flatow EL, Maday MG, Miller SR, McIlveen SJ, Bigliani LU: Open reduction and internal fixation of two- and three-part displaced surgical neck fractures of the proximal humerus. *J Shoulder Elbow Surg* 1992;1:287-295.

20. Hawkins RJ, Bell RH, Gurr K: The three-part fracture of the proximal humerus. *J Bone Joint Surg Am* 1986;68:1410-1414.

21. Sturzenegger M, Fornaro E, Jakob RP: Results of surgical treatment of multifragmented fractures of the proximal humeral head. *Arch Orthop Trauma Surg* 1982;100:249-259.

22. Kunkel SS, Monesmith EA: Isolated avulsion fracture of the lesser tuberosity of the humerus: A case report. *J Shoulder Elbow Surg* 1993;2:43-46.

CHAPTER *4*

HUMERAL HEAD REPLACEMENT ARTHROPLASTY

ANDREW GREEN, MD
STEVEN B. LIPPITT, MD
MICHAEL A. WIRTH, MD

In the 1950s, Neer[1] pioneered the use of humeral head replacement arthroplasty to treat complex proximal humerus fractures. Before then, complex proximal humerus fractures were treated nonsurgically, with open reduction and internal fixation (ORIF), or with humeral head resection. In 1970, Neer[2] proposed and described the four-segment classification system that still is in use. He also reported that ORIF of four-part fractures and fracture-dislocations almost always had unsatisfactory results[3] and recommended humeral head replacement arthroplasty for these injuries. The rationale for arthroplasty was that the injury caused avascularity of the articular segment, which, even with satisfactory reduction and fixation, eventually would collapse, resulting in posttraumatic glenohumeral arthritis and a poor outcome. Humeral head replacement with adequate internal fixation of the tuberosities was believed to provide the best opportunity to achieve a successful outcome.

The principles espoused by Neer in 1970 are still followed. Recent trends in prosthetic replacement for proximal humerus fractures include modular prostheses specifically designed to treat these fractures, improved techniques for tuberosity fixation, and the application of outcome analysis to evaluate the results of this procedure.

ANATOMY

The proximal humerus comprises four major segments: the articular segment, the greater and lesser tuberosities, and the humeral shaft. The muscles that attach to these segments and the magnitude and direction of the forces causing the injury determine the patterns of displacement. In a study of the normal anatomic parameters of the proximal humerus, Iannotti and associates[4] found that the radius of curvature of the average adult humeral head is between 22 and 25 mm and is proportional to the thickness of the humeral head. They also found that the most cephalad surface of the articular segment averages 8 mm above the greater tuberosity. The size of the humeral head determines the lateral displacement of the greater tuberosity and the rotator cuff insertions and affects the kinematics of the glenohumeral joint. Humeral version, another important parameter of humeral anatomy, varies considerably; Pearl and Volk[5] reported a mean retroversion of 29.8 (range, 10° to 55°). These parameters are important for both fracture reconstruction and prosthetic design. Until recently, most prosthetic systems were not designed to precisely reconstruct the normal anatomy of the proximal humerus.

FIGURE 1

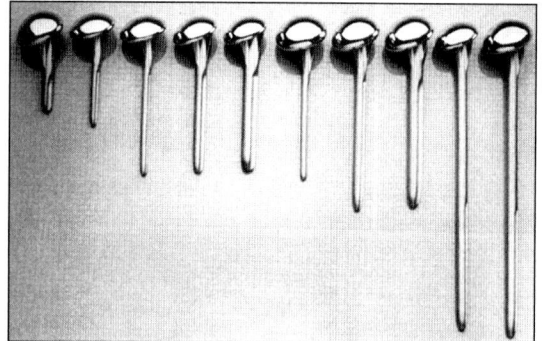

The Neer humeral head prosthesis is a monoblock implant. It has one head radius of curvature and two neck thicknesses. It also has a variety of stem lengths. (Reproduced with permission from Neer CS II: *Shoulder Reconstruction.* Philadelphia, PA, Saunders, 1990.)

FRACTURE CLASSIFICATION AND SURGICAL INDICATIONS

Neer's classification system[2] is based on the four segments of the proximal humerus and emphasizes fracture displacement and its effect on the vascularity of the articular segment. The Comprehensive Long Bone Classification system provides more specific details of fracture patterns but is less widely used.[6] In addition to the identified fracture patterns, other factors such as comminution and osteopenia are important.

Prosthetic arthroplasty is the preferred treatment for most four-part fractures, four-part fracture-dislocations, and head-splitting articular segment fractures. In addition, some three-part fractures are treated with humeral head replacement arthroplasty. Earlier surgery is preferred to reduce the risk of stiffness and heterotopic bone formation. Although some initial reports suggested that surgery be done in the first 48 hours after injury, that is not really necessary, and surgery should be performed as soon as it is feasible. Several studies have demonstrated that the results of primary humeral head replacement for acute proximal humerus fracture are superior to the results of late reconstruction after failed nonsurgical or surgical treatment.[7-9]

IMPLANT DESIGN

The first unconstrained humeral prosthetic designs were monoblock (nonmodular) and did not offer

FIGURE 2

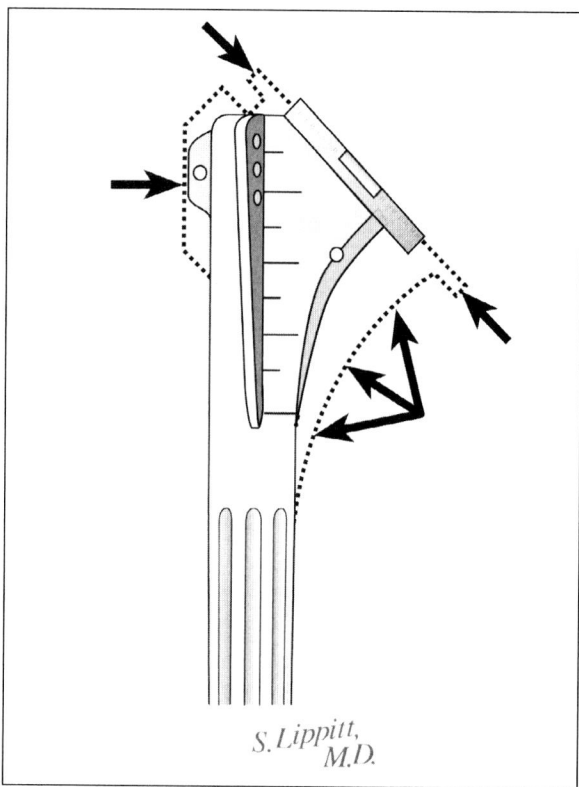

S. Lippitt, M.D.

This diagram shows the difference in the dimensions of the proximal portion of a humeral stem for reconstructive arthroplasty (dashed outline) compared with a prosthesis specifically designed for fracture replacement. The body size of the fracture stem is reduced to facilitate tuberosity reduction without the need to reduce the bony bulk of the tuberosities. *(Copyright © Steven B. Lippitt, MD.)*

variations in humeral head sizes. The first Neer humeral prosthesis had one head radius of curvature and two neck sizes (Figure 1). The second generation of humeral prostheses incorporated modular humeral head replacement. Although the first modular designs provided varying sizes, they were not specifically designed to re-create normal proximal humeral anatomy. Several of the most recent designs specifically address the treatment of fractures. The body size of the stems has been reduced to facilitate tuberosity reduction, and in some systems the humeral head dimensions precisely follow the parameters of normal humeral anatomy (Figure 2). Modular humeral components also potentially facilitate revision surgery.[10,11]

FIGURE 3

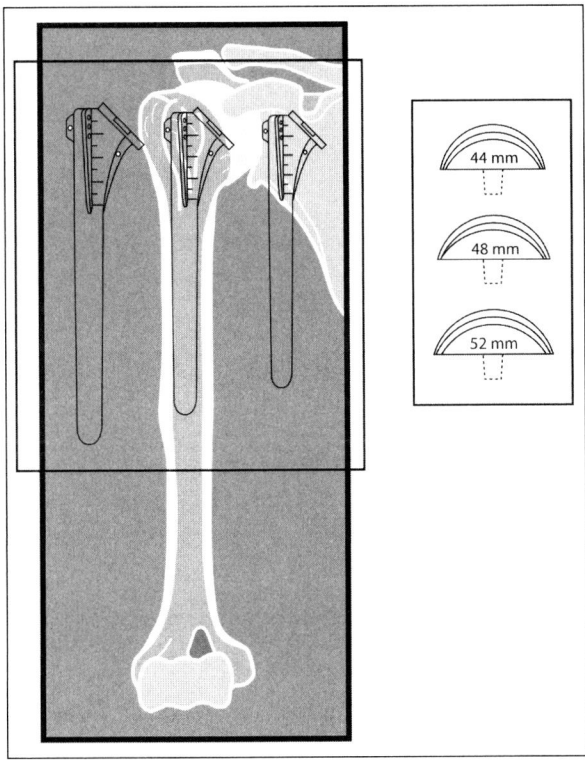

Preoperative templating of radiographs of the contralateral shoulder and humerus can be useful to determine the expected size and position of the humeral component.

SURGICAL TECHNIQUE

Preoperative Evaluation and Planning

Preoperative evaluation and planning are critically important to humeral head replacement for proximal humerus fractures. The general evaluation should include a careful assessment of the patient's neurovascular status, comorbid medical conditions, and psychosocial issues. Swelling and pain can make it difficult to perform a comprehensive neurologic examination. However, a general motor and sensory examination can provide enough information to identify a significant neurologic injury. If the patient's neurologic status remains uncertain, electromyography and nerve conduction velocity studies can be obtained. Nerve injuries are much more commonly associated with proximal humerus fractures and fracture-dislocations than typically reported in studies of humeral head replace-ment.[12,13] de Laat and associates[12] and Visser and associates[13] reported nerve injuries in up to 50% of fractures and fracture-dislocations. Undocumented neurologic injuries probably account for some of the poor results.

Preoperative templating is helpful when planning surgery (Figure 3). Radiographs of the contralateral shoulder can be used to select the expected size and position of the humeral component and are also helpful in late reconstruction.[14]

Technique

Interscalene block regional anesthesia can be used in most patients. Although many patients can undergo surgery with supplemental intravenous anesthesia alone, general anesthesia helps to avoid problems with anxious or restless patients. Either endotracheal or laryngeal mask intubation can be used.

The patient is placed on the operating room table in the beach-chair position, with the arm positioned and supported by a sterile articulating arm holder during the procedure (Figure 4, A). The patient must be far enough over the edge of the table to permit the humerus to be positioned vertically. This position facilitates exposure of the humeral canal for insertion of the prosthesis.

Humeral head replacement is done through a standard deltopectoral approach with a longitudinal incision over the anterior shoulder (Figure 4, B). The incision is begun just superior and lateral to the coracoid and extends toward the anterior aspect of the deltoid insertion. The cephalic vein is preserved and retracted laterally with the deltoid (Figure 4, C). The clavipectoral fascia is incised, and the fracture hematoma is removed. The coracoid should not be osteotomized, and the coracoid muscles are left intact, allowing retraction against the conjoint tendon while protecting the brachial plexus. Abduction of the arm and release of the anterior 1 cm of the deltoid insertion and the upper half of the pectoralis provide more exposure, if necessary, without detachment of the deltoid origin.

Digital palpation is used to identify the axillary nerve inferior to the subscapularis muscle and the musculocutaneous nerve along the deep surface of the coracoid muscles (Figure 4, D and E). The axillary nerve is palpated proximally and distally under the deltoid. When tension is applied to the proximal portion, a pull is felt on the deep deltoid surface. During

FIGURE 4

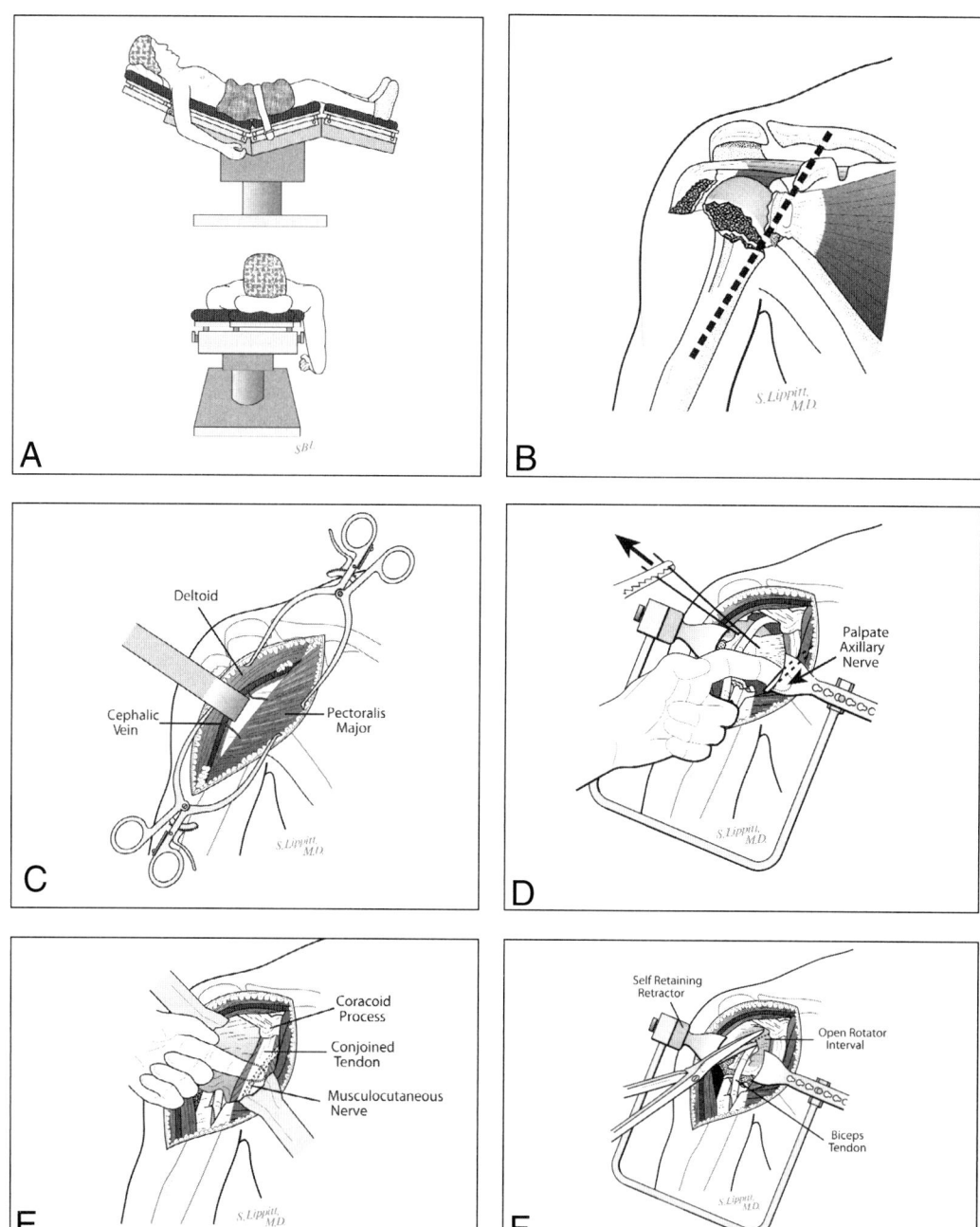

A, The patient is placed in the beach-chair position with the thorax at the edge of the table. This position facilitates vertical positioning of the humerus so that direct access to the medullary canal is unobstructed. **B,** The skin incision is centered over the anterior shoulder and the deltopectoral interval. **C,** The deltopectoral interval is developed, and the cephalic vein is retracted laterally with the deltoid. **D,** The axillary nerve is identified by palpation at the inferior border of the subscapularis muscle. **E,** The musculocutaneous nerve is identified by palpation on the deep surface of the short head of the biceps and coracobrachialis muscles distal to the coracoid process. **F,** The rotator cuff interval is identified by following the long head of the biceps tendon proximally. The interval is opened to separate the greater and lesser tuberosities. *(Copyright © Steven B. Lippitt, MD.)*

surgery, external rotation of the humerus relaxes the tension on the axillary nerve.

If there is an anterior glenohumeral dislocation, the articular segment is identified and removed at this point. Special care must be taken to protect the brachial plexus and peripheral nerves. The articular segment is exposed with careful dissection, the jagged fracture edges are gently freed from surrounding soft tissue, and the humeral head is excised and saved to be used for bone graft.

The tendon of the long head of the biceps, a key anatomic landmark, is identified as it passes under the pectoralis major insertion at the bicipital groove. The transverse humeral ligament is transected, and the biceps tendon is followed to the rotator cuff interval (Figure 4, F). The rotator cuff interval is opened, and the coracohumeral ligament can be released to help mobilize the tuberosities. If the fracture does not involve the bicipital groove, then the groove can be split with an osteotome or saw. If, however, the fracture is adjacent to the groove, it should be left intact, the coracoacromial ligament should not be released, and every effort should be made to preserve the coracoacromial arch. Heavy traction sutures are placed through the rotator cuff insertions on the tuberosities. The articular segment is retrieved and used to select the appropriate size humeral head component.

The glenoid is examined for evidence of articular surface abnormalities, fractures, or labral pathology. A significant glenoid fracture must be stabilized with internal fixation to ensure stability of the glenohumeral joint after replacement. However, if the glenoid cannot be repaired or there is preexisting arthritis, a glenoid component can be used.

The humeral shaft is delivered into the deltopectoral interval by extending the arm off the table and dropping the elbow toward the floor. The surgical neck area is examined for comminution. The medial calcar area is used as a bony landmark for the proper seating of the humeral component. After sizing the humeral shaft by inserting axial reamers into the intramedullary canal, a trial humeral implant is placed with the lateral fin slightly posterior to the bicipital groove and the inferior edge of the medial aspect of the head portion at least at the height of the medial calcar. Packing a sponge into the intramedullary canal helps maintain the position of the implant. Alternatively, some implant systems have fracture jigs to maintain the position of the trial component (Figure 4).

FIGURE 5

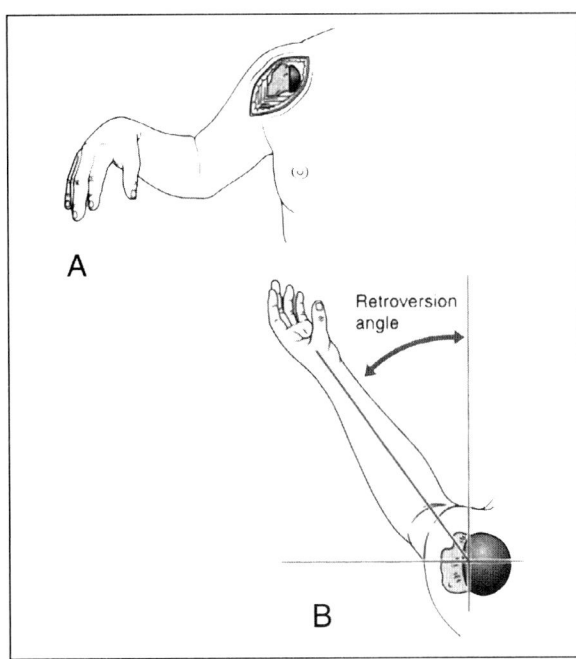

A, Diagram of the upper extremity with the humeral head replacement externally rotated until the flat undersurface of the humeral head is vertically oriented (perpendicular to the floor). **B,** The degree of external rotation is equivalent to the humeral retroversion. (Reproduced with permission from Proximal humeral fractures and glenohumeral dislocation, in Browner BD, et al (eds): *Skeletal Trauma*, ed 2. Philadelphia, PA, Elsevier Science, 2003.)

Humeral Head Version

Several recent studies have demonstrated that humeral head version is variable. Although the mean humeral head retroversion is recognized to be about 30°, retroversion actually varies from approximately 10° to 50°.[5] Ideally, the unique version of each humeral head, which is difficult to determine without referring to a CT scan of the normal side, should be recreated by the surgical reconstruction. Most techniques suggest 30° as a guide for humeral version in fracture replacement. Several techniques are used to determine the humeral version: First, the relationship between the head component and the palpable humeral epicondylar axis is frequently mentioned, but this can be difficult to judge in some patients. Second, the position of the head relative to the externally rotated arm (Figure 5), and third, the position of the fins on the humeral prosthesis can be used to determine the version. The lateral fin of the prosthesis should

FIGURE 6

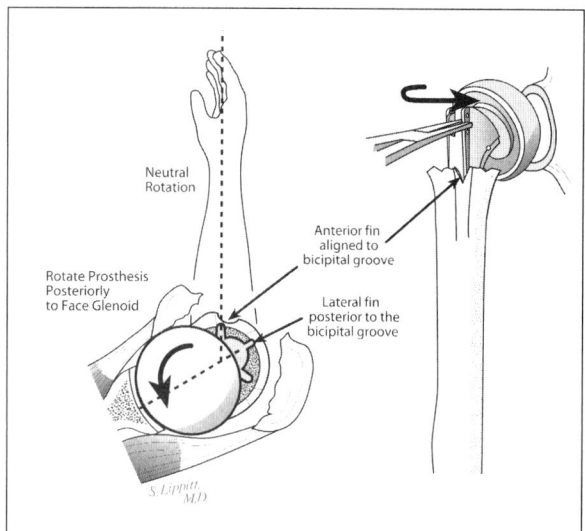

The lateral fin of the humeral component is positioned posterior to the biceps groove. The anterior fin is aligned with the biceps groove. *(Copyright © Steven B. Lippitt, MD.)*

FIGURE 7

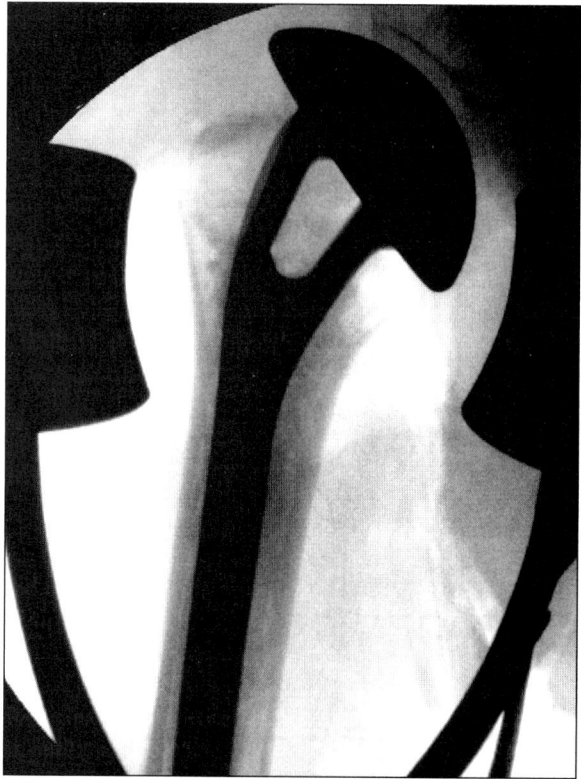

An intraoperative radiograph is used to assess humeral height.

be positioned about 8 mm posterior to the biceps groove (Figure 6). Prosthetic designs that have additional anterior and posterior fins can be positioned so that the anterior fin is aligned with the biceps groove.

Humeral version is an important factor in the reconstruction of the tuberosities.[15] If the humerus is excessively retroverted, there will be increased tension in the greater tuberosity repair, which will limit internal rotation motion and jeopardize the fixation and healing of the greater tuberosity. Conversely, if the humeral component is excessively anteverted, the lesser tuberosity and subscapularis repair may be too tight, risking failure of healing, and external rotation will be limited.

Humeral Head Height

Humeral head height is determined by the position of the humeral head relative to the intact upper end of the humerus. Preoperative templating helps to predict the final position. Tension of the soft tissues, including the deltoid, long head of the biceps, and rotator cuff, can be used to judge the position, and intraoperative imaging is an ideal technique for assessing the humeral head height (Figure 7).

Common errors include removing too much bone and resting the prosthesis too low on the shaft without leaving room for the tuberosities. These errors can result in inferior subluxation of the humeral head because the deltoid myofascial sleeve is rendered too long. Unless the prosthesis restores the humeral length, it will be unstable in the presence of the functionally weakened deltoid.

To prepare the humerus for tuberosity fixation, drill holes are made in the upper shaft so that vertically oriented sutures can be used to repair the tuberosities. A trial reduction is then performed, fitting the mobilized tuberosities with cuff attachments below the level of the articular portion of the component. The tuberosities can be held together with a towel clip while proper head height is determined. A greater tuberosity that is not extensively comminuted can be keyed into place against the upper end of the humerus to identify the appropriate position; however, the correct position and height are more difficult to determine when there is extensive com-

FIGURE 8

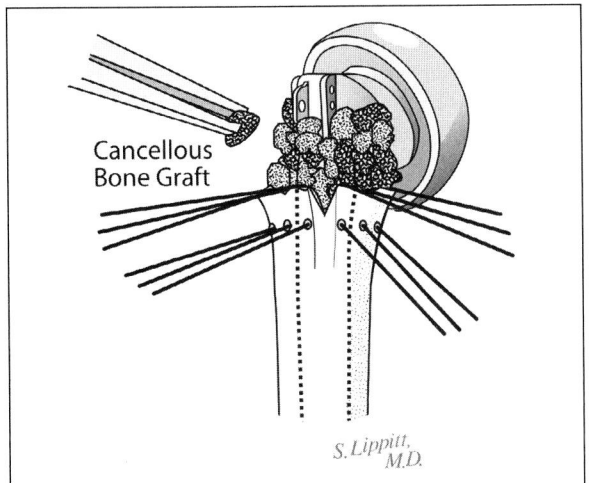

Diagram of a cancellous bone graft placed around the body/metaphyseal portion of the humeral component.

FIGURE 9

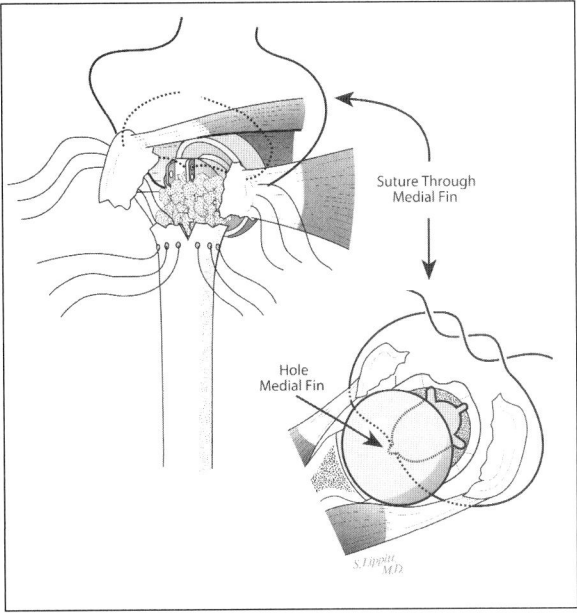

Diagram of circumferentially placed sutures for tuberosity reattachment. *(Copyright © Steven B. Lippitt, MD.)*

minution. In this situation, preoperative templating can be helpful in predicting the appropriate height of the humeral component.

Prosthesis Insertion

The humeral component should be cemented in all fracture patients because it is impossible to predictably achieve an adequate press-fit in these cases. After a cement restrictor is placed to prevent pushing the cement distally, soft polymethylmethacrylate cement is injected into the medullary canal. During cement hardening, excess cement is removed from above the shaft level.

The space between the cemented prosthesis and the shaft is filled by the tuberosities, and autogenous bone graft from the humeral head is packed under the tuberosities and at the tuberosity-shaft juncture to enhance bone healing (Figure 8). Correct reduction of the tuberosities around the humeral implant is important.[15] Many older descriptions of the surgical technique inappropriately depicted positioning the tuberosities around the lateral fin of the humeral implant, which would tend to overtighten the anterior soft tissues. Frankle and associates[15] studied the biomechanics of malposition of the tuberosities and reported that overreduction of the lesser tuberosity around the

humeral implant results in significant impairment of external rotation.

Tuberosity Fixation

Sutures are passed circumferentially around the medial aspect of the prosthesis and the tuberosities for initial tuberosity fixation[16,17] (Figure 9). Frankle and associates[17] demonstrated that circumferential fixation is superior to previously recommended tuberosity-to-tuberosity and tuberosity-to-fin fixation. The sutures around each tuberosity also are passed through the holes in the prosthetic fins, and the vertical sutures in the shaft secure the tuberosities to the shaft. Care is taken to avoid overreducing the tuberosities, the rotator interval is closed, and the repair security, shoulder motion, and stability are evaluated. The limits of motion determined intraoperatively are used to guide postoperative rehabilitation. Generally, there should be close to normal shoulder motion: the glenohumeral joint must be stable to anterior, posterior, and inferior translation, as well as to abduction external rotation and flexion internal rotation. Most authors recommend that there should be 50% posterior translation of the humeral head on the posterior glenoid rim.

The deltopectoral interval is closed. The use of a suction drain is optional and should be based on the appearance of the wound. After subcutaneous and subcuticular skin closure, the arm is placed in a sling unless additional relaxation of the greater tuberosity repair is desirable, in which case, a 45° abduction immobilizer can be used.

Aftercare

Essential aftercare includes ample postoperative support with early physician-guided passive range-of-motion exercises beginning the day after surgery, and active-assisted range-of-motion exercises beginning once early healing has occurred at 6 weeks. Light isometric exercises are added at 6 weeks and isotonic exercises at 12 weeks. At 3 months after surgery most patients should be able to do their regular everyday activities; however, maximal motion and function usually are restored after about 12 months.

RESULTS

Good or excellent results are rarely obtained with nonsurgical treatment of four-part fractures and fracture-dislocations.[18,19] Before the introduction of prosthetic replacement, late treatment of these injuries, with or without head excision, yielded poor results.[20] The results of ORIF for these complex fractures are generally satisfactory in less than 50% of patients.[21-23]

Most authors agree that pain is minimal in more than 90% of patients with prosthetic replacement, and that there are varying results with regard to function, motion, and strength. For example, Green and associates[24] reported 60% excellent and good results and greater than 90% patient satisfaction in a prospective outcome study of humeral head replacement for proximal humerus fractures. In contrast, in Movin and associates'[25] evaluation of 29 proximal humerus fractures treated with humeral head replacement, the results overall were worse than in most other reports, with a mean Constant score of 38. Zyto and associates,[26] after review of 27 patients, were also disappointed with the outcome of hemiarthroplasty because of limited motion and a high incidence of pain and disability.

Becker and associates[27] evaluated the strength and motion of 27 patients with displaced four-part fractures of the proximal humerus treated with hemiarthroplasty. The mean isometric abduction strength was 89% compared with the intact side; mean shoulder abduction was 89° on the operated side and 153° on the intact side ($P < 0.001$). However, despite the significant limitations in strength and motion, 85% of the patients were satisfied with the result.

Factors that affect the outcome of humeral head replacement for fractures have been analyzed in a number of studies.[28-33] These factors include problems with greater tuberosity healing, patient age, timing of surgery, and the quality of the anatomic reconstruction of the proximal humerus.

The position in which the greater tuberosity heals is recognized as one of the most important anatomic factors. Boileau and associates[28] evaluated 66 patients at a mean follow-up of 27 months (range, 18 to 59 months). Of the 33 patients (50%) who had tuberosity malposition at the final evaluation, 18 had initial malposition, and 15 eventually had malposition despite initial correction of positioning. Poor outcome was correlated with tuberosity malposition, superior migration of the humeral prosthesis, stiffness or weakness, persistent pain, poor initial position of the prosthesis (excessive height and/or retroversion), poor position of the greater tuberosity, and women older than age 75 years.[28] Demirhan and associates[34] similarly found that 50% of the complications in their series involved the greater tuberosity and were significantly correlated with poor outcomes. They also reported a significant correlation between outcome and the humeral offset and head height.

Many authors have reported that delay in surgical treatment is associated with inferior clinical outcome.[8,11,35-37] This association seems particularly true when the outcome of acute fracture treatment is compared with the outcome of late reconstruction. Norris and associates[8] reported a retrospective study of 23 patients who had late prosthetic reconstruction of the shoulder after proximal humerus fractures. Although patient satisfaction and pain reduction were predictably satisfactory, functional restoration was variable, and the results were inferior to the authors' experience with primary humeral head replacement for acute proximal humerus fractures. Beredjiklian and associates[35] reported a retrospective study of surgical treatment of 39 patients with malunion of the proximal humerus. Based on criteria of slight or no pain, active elevation greater than 90°, and functional capacity of at least 50% of normal, 69% had a satisfactory result, which was found by the authors to correlate with surgical correction of all osseous and soft-tissue abnormalities. Sperling and associates[36] reported the long-term results of shoulder arthroplasty in patients younger than age 50 years. Of 108 shoulders, 35 had traumatic arthritis; 28 of these were managed with humeral head replacement and seven with total shoulder arthroplasty. The results included 6 excellent (17%), 10 satisfactory (29%), 18 unsatisfactory (51%), and 1 unsuccessful (3%). Boileau and associates[37] reported the largest series of late prosthetic reconstruction after proximal humerus fractures. Using the Constant score, the functional results of the 71 patients they reviewed were 11 excellent (16%), 19 good (26%), 18 average (25%), and 23 poor (33%).

SUMMARY

Acute humeral head replacement is indicated for the treatment of complex proximal humerus fractures when stable internal fixation is not possible or there is considerable risk of fracture-healing complications or posttraumatic osteonecrosis. Recent advances in implant design and surgical technique hold promise for improving the outcome of treatment. Nevertheless, the effects of the traumatic injury and patient selection biases are the likely causes of the poor outcomes. Recognition of associated soft-tissue and neurologic injury is important for the determination of the prognosis for recovery after surgical treatment.

REFERENCES

1. Neer CS II: Articular replacement for the humeral head. *J Bone Joint Surg Am* 1955;37:215-228.
2. Neer CS II: Displaced proximal humeral fractures: I. Classification and evaluation. *J Bone Joint Surg Am* 1970;52:1077-1089.
3. Neer CS II: Displaced proximal humeral fractures: II. Treatment of three-part and four-part displacement. *J Bone Joint Surg Am* 1970;52:1090-1103.
4. Iannotti JP, Gabriel JP, Schneck SL, Evans BG, Misra S: The normal glenohumeral relationships: An anatomical study of one hundred and forty shoulders. *J Bone Joint Surg Am* 1992;74:491-500.
5. Pearl ML, Volk AG: Retroversion of the proximal humerus in relationship to prosthetic replacement arthroplasty. *J Shouler Elbow Surg* 1995;4:286-289.
6. Müller ME, Nazarian S, Koch P, et al: *The Comprehensive Classification of Fractures of Long Bones.* New York, NY, Springer-Verlag, 1990, pp 54-63.
7. Bosch U, Skutek M, Fremery RW, Tscherne H: Outcome after primary and secondary hemiarthroplasty in elderly patients with fractures of the proximal humerus. *J Shoulder Elbow Surg* 1998;7:479-484.
8. Norris TR, Green A, McGuigan FX: Late prosthetic shoulder arthroplasty for displaced proximal humerus fractures. *J Shoulder Elbow Surg* 1995;4:271-280.
9. Tanner MW, Cofield RH: Prosthetic arthroplasty for fractures and fracture-dislocations of the proximal humerus. *Clin Orthop* 1983;179:116-128.
10. Dines DM, Warren RF: Modular shoulder hemiarthroplasty for acute fractures: Surgical considerations. *Clin Orthop* 1994;307:18-26.
11. Moeckel BH, Dines DM, Warren RF, Altchek DW: Modular hemiarthroplasty for fractures of the proximal part of the humerus. *J Bone Joint Surg Am* 1992;74:884-889.
12. de Laat EA, Visser CP, Coene LN, Pahlplatz PV, Tavy DL: Nerve lesions in primary shoulder dislocations and humeral neck fractures: A prospective clinical and EMG study. *J Bone Joint Surg Br* 1994;76:381-383.
13. Visser CP, Tavy DL, Coene LN, Brand R: Electromyographic findings in shoulder dislocations and fractures of the proximal humerus: Comparison with clinical neurological examination. *Clin Neurol Neurosurg* 1999;101:86-91.
14. Green A, Norris TR: Imaging techniques for glenohumeral arthritis and glenohumeral arthroplasty. *Clin Orthop* 1994;307:7-17.
15. Frankle MA, Greenwald DP, Markee BA, Ondrovic LE, Lee WE III: Biomechanical effects of malposition of tuberosity fragments on the humeral prosthetic reconstruction for four-part proximal humerus fractures. *J Shoulder Elbow Surg* 2001;10:321-326.
16. Boileau P, Walch G, Krishnan SG. Tuberosity osteosynthesis and hemiarthroplasty for four part fractures of the proximal humerus. *Tech Shoulder Elbow Surg* 2000;1:96-109.
17. Frankle MA, Ondrovic LE, Markee BA, Harris ML, Lee WE III: Stability of tuberosity reattachment in proximal humeral hemiarthroplasty. *J Shoulder Elbow Surg* 2002;11:413-420.
18. Leyshon R: Closed treatment of fractures of the proximal humerus. *Acta Orthop Scand* 1984;55:48-51.
19. Stableforth PG: Four-part fractures of the neck of the humerus. *J Bone Joint Surg Br* 1984;66:104-108.

20. Neviaser JS: Complicated fractures and dislocations about the shoulder joint. *Instr Course Lect* 1962;44:984-998.

21. Clifford PC: Fractures of the neck of the humerus: A review of the late results. *Injury* 1981;12:91-95.

22. Kristiansen B, Christensen SW: Plate fixation of proximal humeral fractures. *Acta Orthop Scand* 1986;57:320-323.

23. Sturzenegger M, Fornaro E, Jakob RP: Results of surgical treatment of multifragmented fractures of the humeral head. *Arch Orthop Trauma Surg* 1982;100:249-259.

24. Green A, Lippitt SB, Wirth MA: Abstract: Prosthetic hemiarthroplasty for acute proximal humerus fractures: A prospective, multicenter, functional outcomes study. *65th Annual Meeting Proceedings*. Rosemont, IL, American Academy of Orthopaedic Surgeons, 1998, p 205.

25. Movin T, Sjödén GOJ, Ahrengart L: Poor function after shoulder replacement in fracture patients: A retrospective evaluation of 29 patients followed for 2-12 years. *Acta Orthop Scand* 1998;69:392-396.

26. Zyto K, Wallace WA, Frostick SP, Preston BJ: Outcome after hemiarthroplasty for three-and four-part fractures of the proximal humerus. *J Shoulder Elbow Surg* 1998;7:85-89.

27. Becker R, Pap G, Machner A, Neumann WH: Strength and motion after hemiarthroplasty in displaced four-fragment fracture of the proximal humerus: 27 patients followed for 1-6 years. *Acta Orthop Scand* 2002;73:44-49.

28. Boileau P, Krishnan SG, Tinsi L, Walch G, Coste JS, Mole D: Tuberosity malposition and migration: Reasons for poor outcomes after hemiarthroplasty for displaced fractures of the proximal humerus. *J Shoulder Elbow Surg* 2002;11:401-412.

29. Goldman RT, Koval KJ, Cuomo F, Gallagher MA, Zuckerman JD: Functional outcome after humeral head replacement for acute three- and four-part proximal humerus fractures. *J Shoulder Elbow Surg* 1995;4:81-86.

30. Green A, Barnard WL, Limbird RS: Humeral head replacement for acute, four-part proximal humerus fractures. *J Shoulder Elbow Surg* 1993;2:249-254.

31. Hawkins RJ, Switlyk P: Acute prosthetic replacement for severe fractures of the proximal humerus. *Clin Orthop* 1993;289:156-160.

32. Kay SP, Amstutz HC: Shoulder hemiarthroplasty at UCLA. *Clin Orthop* 1988;228:42-48.

33. Wretenberg P, Ekelund A: Acute hemiarthroplasty after proximal humerus fracture in old patients: A retrospective evaluation of 18 patients followed for 2-7 years. *Acta Orthop Scand* 1997;68:121-123.

34. Demirhan M, Kilicoglu O, Altinel L, Eralp L, Akalin Y: Prognostic factors in prosthetic replacement for acute proximal humerus fractures. *J Orthop Trauma* 2003;17:181-189.

35. Beredjiklian PK, Iannotti JP, Norris TR, Williams GR: Operative treatment of malunion of a fracture of the proximal aspect of the humerus. *J Bone Joint Surg Am* 1998;80:1484-1497.

36. Sperling JW, Cofield RH, Rowland CM: Neer hemiarthroplasty and Neer total shoulder arthroplasty in patients fifty years old or less: Long-term results. *J Bone Joint Surg Am* 1998;80:464-473.

37. Boileau P, Walch G, Trojani C, Sinnerton R, Romeo AA, Veneau B: Sequelae of fractures of the proximal humerus: Surgical classification and limits of shoulder arthroplasty, in Walch G, Boileau P (eds): *Shoulder Arthroplasty*. Berlin, Germany, Springer-Verlag, 1999, pp 349-358.

CHAPTER 5

LATE SEQUELAE OF PROXIMAL HUMERUS FRACTURES

MICHAEL A. WIRTH, MD

Fractures of the proximal humerus account for 4% to 5% of all fractures.[1,2] Approximately 60% to 80% of these injuries are minimally displaced (a so-called one-part fracture) and can be satisfactorily treated with a sling and early range-of-motion exercises. Contrary to popular belief, the seemingly innocuous nature of these minimally displaced fractures does not preclude the development of complications. In general, late sequelae of proximal humerus fractures include refractory shoulder stiffness, osteonecrosis, malunion, nonunion, and heterotopic bone formation. The aftereffects of both minimally displaced and more complex multiple-part proximal humerus fractures may result from the injury itself or the treatment. Consequently, it is imperative to make an accurate diagnosis so that the most appropriate treatment can be instituted in a timely fashion (Figure 1).

REFRACTORY SHOULDER STIFFNESS

Shoulder stiffness is one of the most common aftereffects of proximal humerus fractures. Factors that

contribute to this complication include the severity of the initial injury, prolonged immobilization, articular surface malunion, and noncompliance with rehabilitation. In a functional outcome study of 104 patients with minimally displaced proximal humerus fractures, the percentage of good and excellent results was significantly greater when supervised physical therapy was initiated less than 14 days after injury.[3] Shoulder stiffness also has a negative effect on displaced three- and four-part proximal humerus fractures. The outcome of late arthroplasty for these complex fractures is inferior to that of acute humeral head replacement, largely as a result of fixed soft tissue.[4-6] Numerous studies have emphasized the importance of an early physician-directed rehabilitation program for both nonsurgically and surgically managed patients in an effort to minimize refractory shoulder stiffness.[7-10]

OSTEONECROSIS

The incidence of osteonecrosis generally is proportional to the complexity of the proximal humerus frac-

FIGURE 1

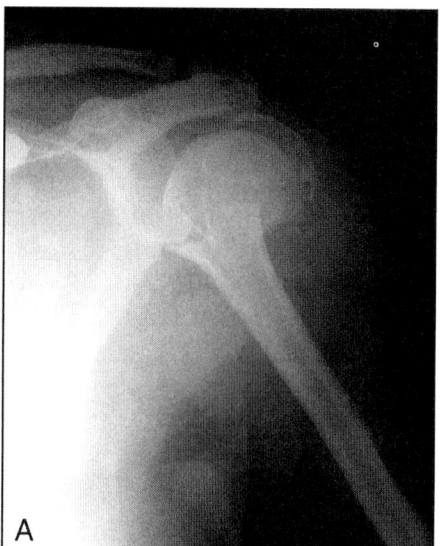 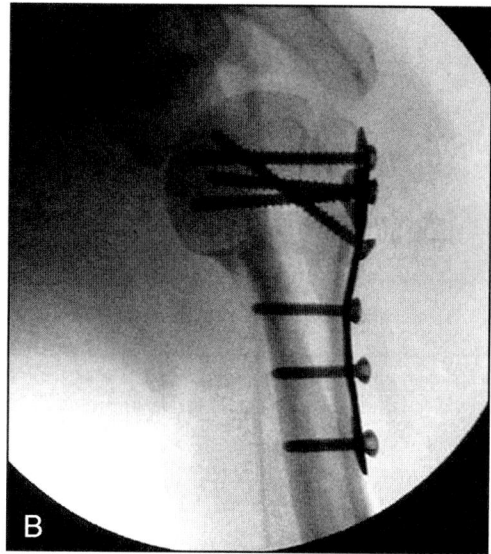

A and **B**, Three-part proximal humerus fracture treated with ORIF. Passive range-of-motion exercises were begun on the first postoperative day with excellent return to function.

FIGURE 2

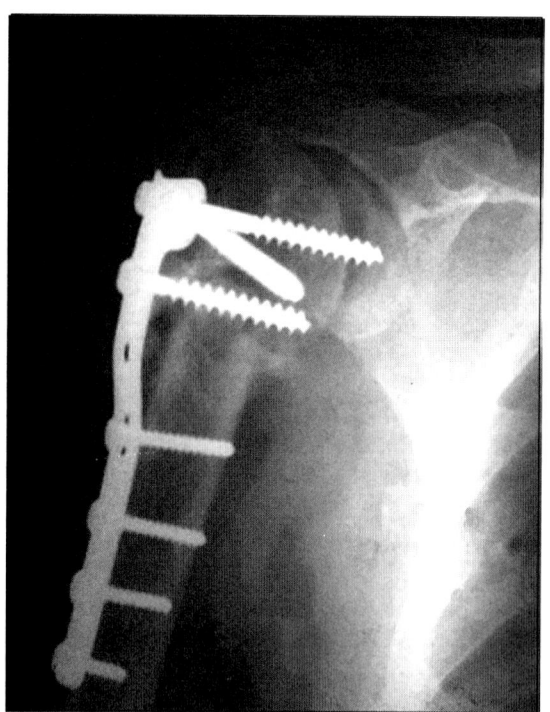

Postoperative AP radiograph showing an excessively long cancellous fixation screw that penetrated the glenohumeral joint.

ture, the extent of surgical dissection of the soft tissue, and additional surgeon-controlled variables. Complications can be minimized with careful preoperative planning and a thorough understanding of three-dimensional anatomy. For example, lack of familiarity with the geometry of the humeral head during open reduction and internal fixation (ORIF) may result in penetration of the humeral head articular surface while drilling (Figure 2), which may cause chondrolysis of the humeral head and ultimately lead to glenohumeral arthritis. Osteonecrosis usually is associated with three- and four-part fractures and fracture-dislocations and only rarely with two-part fractures. The prevalence ranges from 3% to 14% after closed reduction of displaced three-part fractures and from 13% to 34% after reduction of four-part fractures.[11-18] Sturzenegger and associates[19] reported a 34% incidence of osteonecrosis in a series of patients treated with ORIF with a T-plate. The pathology may be detected by MRI before it is seen with conventional radiography. Later, osteoporosis or osteosclerosis may be seen on plain radio-graphs. In end-stage osteonecrosis, collapse of the subchondral bone occurs, and eventually, the irregular humeral head destroys the glenoid articular cartilage and results in secondary degenerative joint disease (Figure 3). Pros-

FIGURE 3

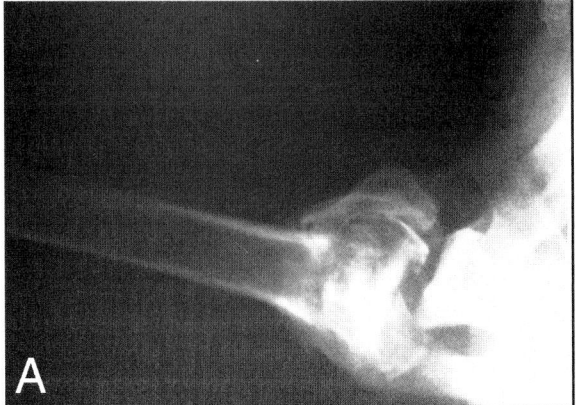

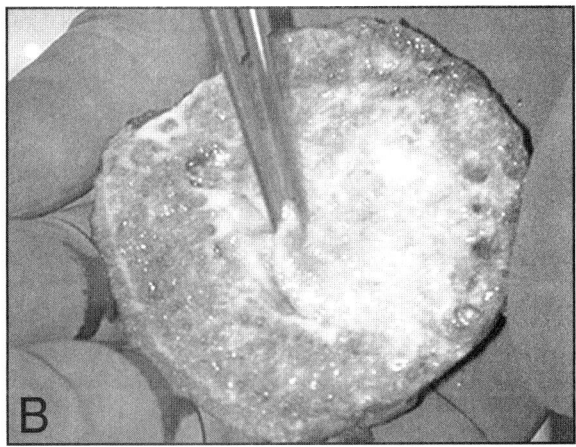

A, Axillary lateral radiograph revealing osteonecrosis of the humeral head associated with degenerative changes of the shoulder joint. **B**, Intraoperative photograph of the resected humeral head during total shoulder arthroplasty.

thetic arthroplasty is the primary surgical option in the presence of severe pain and functional loss.

MALUNION

Malunion results when closed reduction or failed ORIF does not restore the normal anatomic relationships between the humeral head and shaft, tuberosities, and glenohumeral joint (Figure 4). Malunion of the greater tuberosity is usually superior and/or posterior. Superior displacement that encroaches on the subacromial space will result in

FIGURE 4

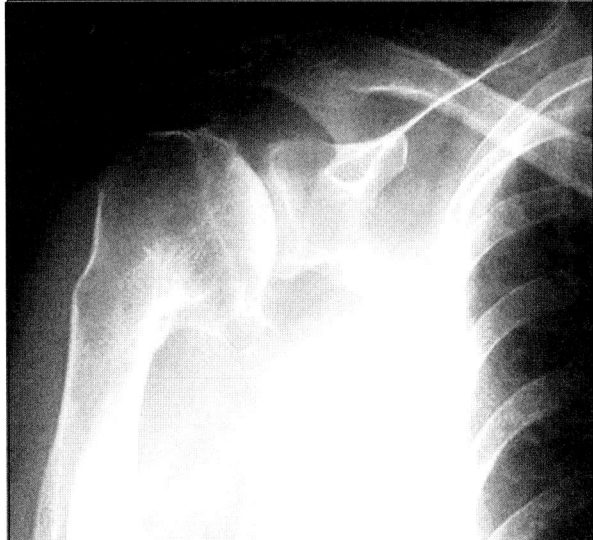

Malunion of the proximal humerus. Note the distorted appearance of the proximal humeral geometry.

pain, weakness, and a mechanical block to overhead elevation (Figure 5); predominantly posterior displacement limits external rotation because of abutment with the posterior glenoid. When pain and functional limitations are present, osteotomy is indicated if displacement exceeds 5 mm. Fixed soft-tissue contractures make it difficult to adequately immobilize and fix the tuberosity in a fashion that restores the dynamic quality of the rotator cuff muscle-tendon unit. Thorough preoperative counseling to discuss reasonable expectations is essential because functional results often are modest.

Two-part surgical neck fractures rarely result in pain or functional limitation that would necessitate surgical intervention. Occasionally, a varus malunion causes impingement between the acromion and the superiorly displaced greater tuberosity. In many patients, varus malunion can be treated adequately by open or arthroscopic acromioplasty with or without a greater tuberosity. Humeral head articular malunions associated with joint incongruity and subsequent degenerative changes result from malunited three- and four-part proximal humerus fractures. Prosthetic arthroplasty is generally required for this type of late

FIGURE 5

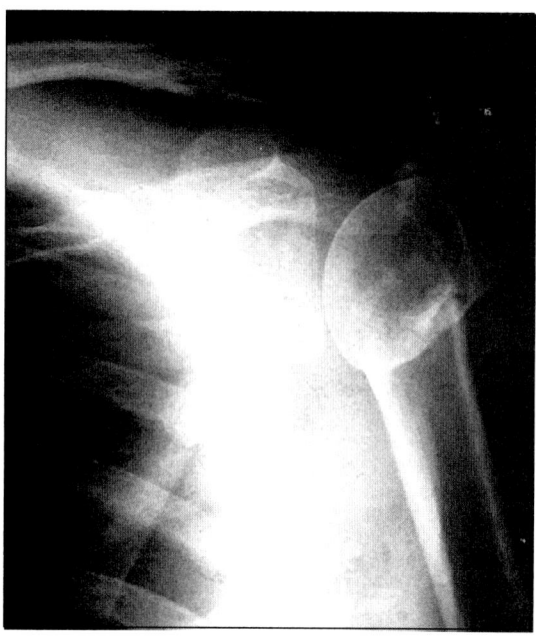

Superior displacement of this greater tuberosity malunion resulted in a functional loss of abduction and elevation.

FIGURE 6

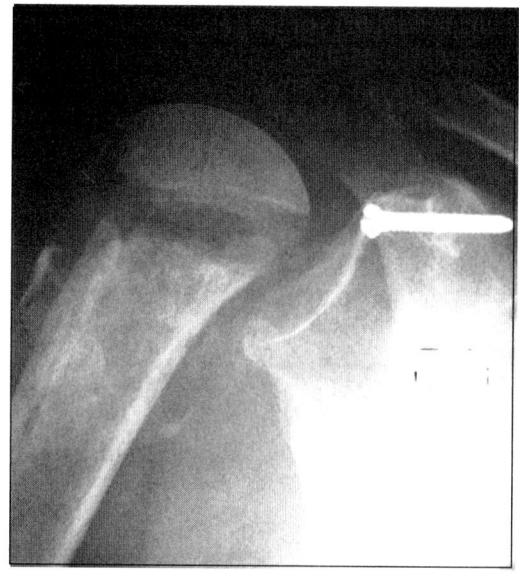

Initial surgical management included nonrigid ORIF. Note the valgus position of the humeral head nonunion and resorption of the greater and lesser tuberosities.

sequela. Extensive scarring, deltoid weakness, inferior pain relief, and a higher incidence of complications result in a less favorable prognosis than for fractures managed acutely.

NONUNION

Nonunion of the proximal humerus occurs most commonly in elderly patients with osteoporosis.[20-23] The incidence of this late sequela is difficult to determine, but it may occur in up to 23% of surgical neck fractures in the elderly[24] (Figure 6). Factors associated with nonunion of the proximal humerus include soft-tissue interposition, hanging arm casts, inadequate ORIF, alcoholism, and comorbidities such as diabetes mellitus.[25-32] In many patients the nonunion is associated with minimal pain and a functional range of motion that obviates the need for surgery.[33-41] Closed methods of treatment that require prolonged immobilization or extremes of positioning are inappropriate because they can result in functionally disabling arthrofibrosis.

Surgical treatment options for patients with pain

FIGURE 7

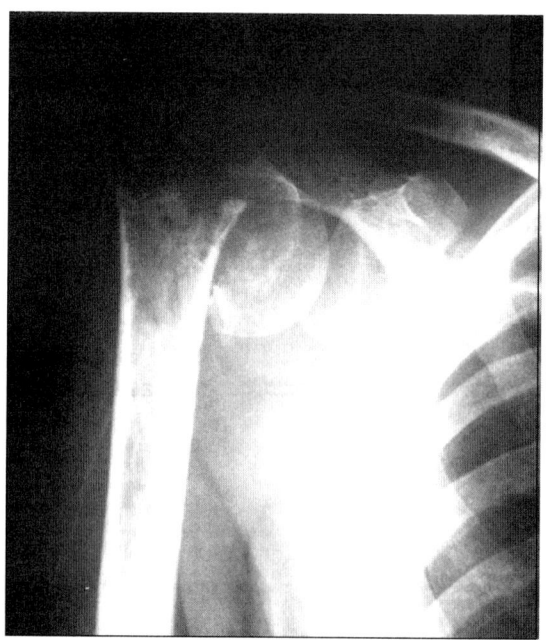

Proximal humerus nonunion associated with loss of cancellous bone from the humeral head.

FIGURE 8

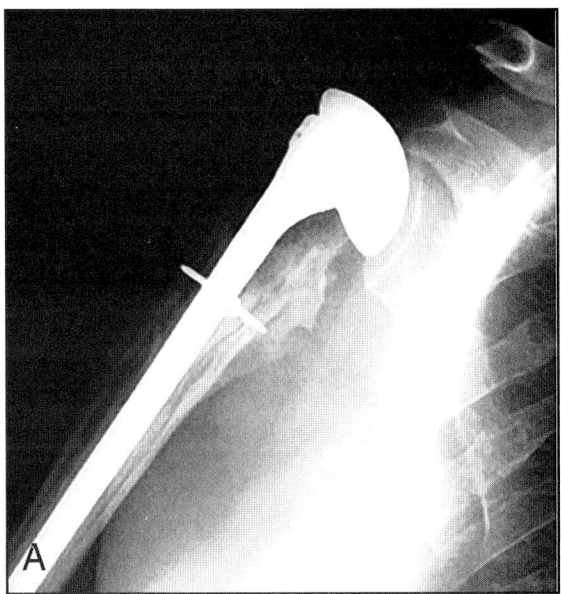
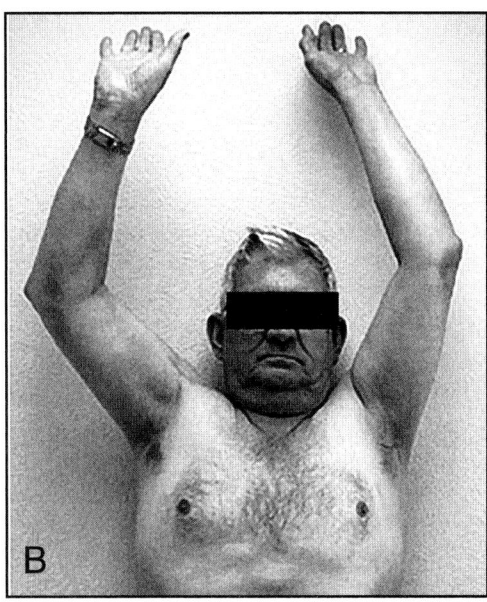

A, AP radiograph of the right shoulder demonstrating heterotopic bone formation following surgery. **B,** Elevation at 6 months after surgery.

and functional disability are based largely on the quality of the bone, the stability of the surgical construct at the time of the operation, the integrity of the humeral head and glenoid articular surfaces, and the vascularity of the humeral head. ORIF with bone grafting is the preferred method of treatment when adequate bone quality and quantity allow secure fixation that permits early rehabilitation while avoiding the complications associated with prolonged immobilization. Unfortunately, many surgical neck nonunions are associated with resorption of the humeral head fragment and cavitation, resulting in severe bone loss (Figure 7).

HETEROTOPIC BONE FORMATION

The formation of ectopic bone about the proximal humerus following fracture is common and, in most cases, clinical relevance to the patient's functional outcome is minimal.[42-44] In 1970, Neer[43] described a series of 117 consecutive patients with three- and four-part fractures and fracture-dislocations. Ectopic ossification occurred in 12% of the patients, including three patients managed with closed reduction, five

treated with ORIF, and six who underwent hemiarthroplasty. The extent of soft-tissue injury, repeated manipulation, and delayed reduction beyond 7 days were considered predisposing factors. In most patients, ectopic bone formation represents an incidental radiographic finding (Figure 8). Only rarely does the bone formation bridge the glenohumeral space and result in limited motion. In this situation, surgical resection is indicated to restore a functional range of motion after radioisotope imaging reveals normal cellular activity.

REFERENCES

1. Lind T, Kroner K, Jensen J: The epidemiology of fractures of the proximal humerus. *Arch Orthop Trauma Surg* 1989;108:285-287.

2. Stimson BB: *A Manual of Fractures and Dislocations*, ed 2. Philadelphia, PA, Lea and Febiger, 1947, pp 241-260.

3. Koval K, Gallagher MA, Maroicano JG, Cuomo F, McShinawy A, Zuckerman JD: Functional outcome after minimally displaced fractures of the proximal part of the humerus. *J Bone Joint Surgery Am* 1997;79:203-207.

4. Frisch LH, Sojberg JO, Sneppen O: Shoulder arthroplasty in complex acute and chronic proximal humeral fractures. *Orthopedics* 1991;9:949-954.

5. Neer CS II: Glenohumeral arthroplasty, in Neer CS II (ed): *Shoulder Reconstruction.* Philadelphia, PA, WB Saunders, 1990, pp 143-269.

6. Tanner MW, Cofield RH: Prosthetic arthroplasty for fractures and fracture-dislocations of the proximal humerus. *Clin Orthop* 1983;179:116-128.

7. Bertoft ES, Lundh I, Ringqvist I: Physiotherapy after fracture of the proximal end of the humerus. *Scand J Rehabil Med* 1984;16:11-16.

8. Brostrom F: Early mobilization of fractures of the upper end of the humerus. *Arch Surg* 1943;46:614.

9. Ekstrom T, Lagergren C, Von Schreeb T: Procaine injections and early mobilization for the fractures of the neck of the humerus. *Acta Chir Scand* 1965;130:18-24.

10. Gristina AG: Management of displaced fractures of the proximal humerus. *Contemp Orthop* 1987;15:61-93.

11. Fournier P, Martini M: Post-traumatic avascular necrosis of the humeral head. *Int Orthop* 1977;1:187-190.

12. Geneste R, Durandeau A, Gauzere JM, Roy J: The treatment of fracture-dislocation of the humeral head by blind pinning. *Rev Chir Orthop Reparatrice Appar Mot* 1980;66:383-386.

13. Hagg O, Lundberg B: Aspects of prognostic factors in comminuted and dislocated proximal humeral fractures, in Bateman JE, Welsh RP (eds): *Surgery of the Shoulder.* Philadelphia, PA, BC Decker, 1984, pp 51-59.

14. Jakob RP, Kristiansens T, Mayo K, Ganz R, Muller ME: Classification and aspects of treatment of fractures of the proximal humerus, in Bateman JE, Welsh RP (eds): *Surgery of the Shoulder.* Philadelphia, PA, BC Decker, 1984.

15. Knight RA, Mayne JA: Comminuted fractures and fracture-dislocations involving the articular surface of the humeral head. *J Bone Joint Surg Am* 1957;39:1343-1355.

16. Kristiansen B, Christensen SW: Plate fixation of proximal humeral fractures. *Acta Orthop Scand* 1986;57:320-323.

17. Lee CK, Hansen HR: Post-traumatic avascular necrosis of the humeral head in displaced proximal humeral fractures. *J Trauma* 1981;21:788-791.

18. Wirth M, Jensen K, Agarwal A, Curtis R, Rockwood C Jr: Fracture dislocation of the proximal part of the humerus with retroperitoneal displacement of the humeral head. *J Bone Joint Surg Am* 1997;79:763-766.

19. Sturzenegger M, Fornaro E, Jakob RP: Results of surgical treatment of multifragmented fractures of the humeral head. *Arch Orthop Trauma Surg* 1982;100:249-259.

20. Rose SH, Melton LJ III, Morrey BF, et al: Epidemiologic features of humeral fractures. *Clin Orthop* 1982;168:24-30.

21. Neer CS II: Displaced proximal humeral fractures: I. Classification and evaluation. *J Bone Joint Surg Am* 1970;52:1077-1089.

22. Neer CS II: Four-segment classification of displaced proximal humeral fractures. *Instr Course Lect* 1975;24:160-168.

23. Sorensen KH: Pseudoarthrosis of the surgical neck of the humerus: Two cases, one bilateral. *Acta Orthop Scand* 1964;34:132-138.

24. Neer CS II: Non-union of the surgical neck of the humerus. *Orthop Trans* 1983;7:389.

25. Coventry MB, Laurnen EL: Ununited fractures of the middle and upper humerus: Special problems in treatment. *Clin Orthop* 1970;69:192-198.

26. Ray RD, Sankaran B, Fetrow KO: Delayed union and non-union of fractures. *J Bone Joint Surg Am* 1964;46:627-643.

27. Rooney PJ, Cockshott WP: Pseudoarthrosis following proximal humeral fractures: A possible mechanism. *Skeletal Radiol* 1986;15:21-24.

28. Epps CH Jr, Cotler JM: Complications of treatment of fractures of the humeral shaft, in Epps CH Jr (ed): *Complications in Orthopaedic Surgery*, ed 2. Philadelphia, PA, JB Lippincott, 1986, pp 277-304.

29. Mayer PJ, Evarts CM: Nonunion, delayed union, malunion, and avascular necrosis, in Epps CH Jr (ed.): *Complications in Orthopaedic Surgery*, ed 2. Philadelphia, PA, JB Lippincott, 1986, pp 207-230.

30. Muller ME, Thomas RJ: Treatment of non-union in fractures of long bones. *Clin Orthop* 1979;138:141-153.

31. Neviasier JS: Complicated fractures and dislocations about the shoulder joint. *J Bone Joint Surg Am* 1962;44:984-998.

32. Paavolainen, P, Bjorkenheim JM, Slatis P, et al: Operative treatment of severe proximal humeral fractures. *Acta Orthop Scand* 1983; 54:374-379.

33. Leach RE, Premer RF: Nonunion of the surgical neck of the humerus: Method of internal fixation. *Minn Med* 1965;48:318-322.

34. Neer CS II: Fractures and dislocations of the shoulder: Part I. Fractures about the shoulder, in Rockwood CA Jr, Green DP (eds): *Fractures in Adults*, ed 2. Philadelphia, PA, JB Lippincott, 1984, pp 675-721.

35. DePalma AF, Cautilli RA. Fractures of the upper end of the humerus. *Clin Orthop* 1961;20:73-93.

36. Dingeley A, Denham R: Fracture-dislocation of the humeral head: A method of reduction. *J Bone Joint Surg Am* 1973;55:1299-1300.

37. Drapanas T, McDonald J, Hale HW Jr: A rational approach to classification and treatment of fractures of the surgical neck of the humerus. *Am J Surg* 1960;99:617- 624.

38. Keene JS, Huizengia RE, Engber WD, et al: Proximal humeral fractures: A correlation of residual deformity with long-term function. *Orthopedics* 1983;6:173-178.

39. Perkins G: Rest and movement. *J Bone Joint Surg Br* 1953;35:521-539.

40. Young TB, Wallace WA: Conservation treatment of fractures and fracture-dislocations of the upper end of the humerus. *J Bone Joint Surg Br* 1985;67:373-377.

41. Laing PG: The arterial supply of the adult humerus. *J Bone Joint Surg Am* 1956;38:1105-1116.

42. Wirth MA, Rockwood CA Jr: Complications of shoulder arthroplasty. *Clin Orthop* 1993;307;47-69.

43. Neer CS: Displaced proximal humeral fractures: II. Treatment of three-part and four-part displacement. *J Bone Joint Surg Am* 1970;52:1090-1103.

44. Wirth MA, Rockwood CA Jr: Complications of total shoulder replacement arthroplasty. *J Bone Joint Surg Am* 1996;78:603-616.

INDEX